Pediatric Treatm‹

New AAP Guidelines

2004 Edition

Karen Scruggs, MD

Michael T. Johnson, MD

Current Clinical Strategies Publishing

www.ccspublishing.com/ccs

Digital Book and Updates

Purchasers of this book may download the digital book and updates for Palm, Pocket PC, Windows and Macintosh. The digital books can be downloaded at the Current Clinical Strategies Publishing Internet site:

www.ccspublishing.com/ccs/pedtreat.htm

Current Clinical Strategies Publishing
27071 Cabot Road
Laguna Hills, California 92653
Phone: 800-331-8227
Fax: 800-965-9420
info@ccspublishing.com
Internet: www.ccspublishing.com/ccs

Printed in USA

ISBN 1-929622-26-0

Contents

Neonatology

Normal Newborn Care

I. Prenatal pediatric visit

A. The prenatal pediatric visit usually takes place during the third trimester of the pregnancy. Maternal nutrition, the hazards of alcohol, cigarette smoking and other drugs, and the dangers of passive smoking should be discussed. Maternal illnesses and medications should be reviewed.

Prenatal Pediatric Visit Discussion Issues

Maternal History
  General health and nutrition
  Past and present obstetric history
  Maternal smoking, alcohol, or drug use
  Maternal medications
  Infectious diseases: Hepatitis, herpes, syphilis, Chlamydia rubella
  Maternal blood type and Rh blood groups
Family History
Newborn Issues
  Assessment of basic parenting skills
  Feeding plan: Breast feeding vs formula
  Car seats
  Circumcision of male infant

II. Delivery

A. Neonatal resuscitation

1. All equipment must be set up and checked before delivery. The infant who fails to breath spontaneously at birth should be placed under a radiant warmer, dried, and positioned to open the airway. The mouth and nares should be suctioned, and gentle stimulation provided.

2. The mouth should be suctioned first to prevent aspiration. Prolonged or overly vigorous suctioning may lead to bradycardia and should be avoided unless moderate-to-thick meconium is present in the airway.

3. The infant born with primary apnea is most likely to respond to the stimulation of drying and gentle tapping of the soles of the feet. The infant who fails to respond rapidly to these measures is experiencing secondary apnea and requires positive pressure bag ventilation with oxygen.

4. Adequate ventilation is assessed by looking for chest wall excursions and listening for air exchange. The heart rate should be assessed while positive pressure ventilation is being applied. If the heart rate does not increase rapidly after ventilation, chest compressions must be started by an assistant. If the infant fails to respond to these measures, intubation and medications are necessary. Epinephrine can be administered via the endotracheal tube. Apgar scores are used to assess the status of the infant at 1 and 5 min following delivery.

Apgar Scoring System			
Sign	0	1	2
Heart rate	Absent	Slow (<100 beats/min)	100 beats/min or more
Respirations	Absent	Weak cry; hypoventilation	Strong cry
Muscle tone	Limp	Some flexion	Active motion
Reflex irritability	No response	Grimace	Cough or sneeze
Color	Blue or pale	Body pink; extremities blue	Completely pink

III. **Early routine care of the newborn**
   A. **Vitamin K** is given to the infant by intramuscular injection to prevent hemorrhagic disease of the newborn.
   B. **Ocular prophylaxis** against gonorrheal and chlamydial infection is administered after birth with erythromycin ophthalmic ointment.
   C. **Umbilical cord blood syphilis serology** is completed if there is no documented record of a negative third-trimester maternal test. Umbilical cord care consists of local application of triple dye or bacitracin ointment.
   D. **Hepatitis B prophylaxis**. If the mother is hepatitis B surface antigen-positive, or if she has active hepatitis B, the infant should be given an IM injection of hepatitis B immune globulin and a course of three injections of hepatitis B vaccine (before hospital discharge, and at 1 and 6 months of age).

IV. **Physical examination of the newborn**
   A. **General gestalt**. The examiner should assess whether the infant appears to be sick or well. An unusual cry may indicate sepsis, hypothyroidism, a congenital anomaly of the larynx, or a chromosomal abnormality.
   B. **Vital signs**. The normal temperature of the newborn is 36.5 to 37.0 degrees C. The normal respiratory rate ranges from 40 to 60 breaths per minute, and the normal heart rate can range from 94 to 175 beats per minute.
   C. **Assessment of the adequacy of fetal growth**
      1. **Gestational age assessment.** The gestational age of the newborn infant is assessed with the Ballard score of neuromuscular and physical maturity.
      2. **Premature infants**
         a. A preterm infant is defined as an infant of less than 37 weeks' gestation, and a postterm infant is defined as being of greater than 42 weeks' gestation.
         b. Preterm infants may develop respiratory distress syndrome, apnea, bradycardia, and retinopathy of prematurity. Respiratory distress syndrome is recognized by tachypnea, grunting, retractions, an elevated oxygen requirement, and a roentgenographic picture of poor inflation and a fine homogeneous ground-glass appearance.
   D. **Premature infants** of less than 34-1/2 to 35 weeks' gestation are at increased risk for apnea and bradycardia. Apnea is defined as a respiratory pause of 20 sec or longer and frequently is accompanied by a drop in heart rate.

E. Measurements and growth charts

1. Height, weight, and head circumference should be measured. A low-birth-weight infant is defined as any neonate with a birthweight <2,500 g. Height, weight, and head circumference should be plotted as a function of gestational age on an intrauterine growth chart.

2. Factors that may result in an infant who is small for gestational age include chromosomal and other dysmorphic syndromes, congenital infections, maternal hypertension, smoking, uterine anomalies, and multiple gestations.

3. The small-for-gestational age infant is at greater risk for cold stress, hypoglycemia, hypocalcemia, and polycythemia.

4. The differential diagnosis for the large-for-gestational age infant includes maternal diabetes and maternal obesity. The large-for-gestational age infant is at risk for shoulder dystocia, birth trauma, and hypoglycemia.

F. Examination of organ systems and regions

1. **Head, face, and neck**
   a. **The head circumference** is measured and plotted, and the scalp, fontanelles, and sutures are examined. Bruising and hematomas of the scalp should be noted. Cephalohematomas are subperiosteal and do not cross suture lines, whereas caputs are subcutaneous and do cross suture lines.
   b. **Facial features** that suggest a chromosomal anomaly include midfacial hypoplasia, small eyes, or low-set ears. Fetal alcohol syndrome is suggested by a small upper lip and a smooth philtrum.
   c. **The eyes** should be examined with an ophthalmoscope to document a red reflex. The absence of a clear red reflex is indicative of a retinoblastoma, cataract, or glaucoma.
   d. **The lips, mouth, and palate** are inspected and palpated for clefts. **Nares patency** can be documented by closing the mouth and occluding one nostril at a time while observing air flow through the opposite nostril.

2. **Thorax and cardiovascular systems**
   a. **Chest wall excursions** should be observed and the respiratory rate determined. The normal neonatal respiratory rate is 40 to 60 breaths per minute.
   b. **Auscultation of breath and heart sounds.** The normal heart rate during the first week of life may range from 94 to 175 beats per minute.

3. **Abdomen and gastrointestinal system**
   a. **Visual inspection of the abdomen** should assess symmetry and distension.
   b. **Abdominal palpation** for masses, hepatosplenomegaly, or renal masses is completed, and the anus should be visually inspected.

4. **Genitourinary system.** The genitalia are examined for ambiguous genitalia, which requires immediate endocrinologic and urologic consultation.

5. **Musculoskeletal system**
   a. **Hip examination** may detect developmental dysplasia. Risk factors for hip dysplasia include a family history, foot deformities, congenital torticollis, Down syndrome, and breech presentation. The female to male ratio is 7:1. Ultrasonography is used to evaluate suspected hip dysplasia.
   b. **Fracture of the clavicle** occurs in 0.2-3.5% of vaginal deliveries. Physical findings include local swelling and crepitations and an asymmetric Moro reflex. Treatment consists of making a sling by pinning the shirt sleeve of the involved side to the opposite side of the shirt.

6. **Neurologic system**
   a. The degree of alertness, activity, and muscle tone should be noted. The head circumference is plotted on the growth chart.
   b. The posterior midline area should be examined for evidence of neural tube defects. Pilonidal dimples with tufts of hair are evaluated with ultrasonography.

V. Common neonatal problems
A. Hypoglycemia
1. Hypoglycemia is common in premature infants, infants who are small for gestational age, infants of diabetic mothers, and infants who have experienced perinatal asphyxia.
2. Hypoglycemia is defined as a blood glucose of <40-45 mg/dL. Hypoglycemic infants require early feedings or IV glucose.

B. Anemia during the newborn period may be caused by hemolytic and congenital anemias, fetal-to-maternal hemorrhage, placental abruption, and occult hemorrhage.

C. Bilirubin metabolism
1. Hyperbilirubinemia occurs frequently in the normal newborn because of increased production and decreased elimination of this breakdown product of heme.
2. Initial workup for neonatal hyperbilirubinemia includes measurements of total and direct bilirubin levels, hematocrit, Coombs test, and testing of urine for reducing substances to exclude galactosemia. High levels of bilirubin can cause an acute encephalopathy (ie, kernicterus).

D. Gastrointestinal problems
1. Ninety-six percent of full-term newborns pass a meconium stool before 24 hours of age. A delayed or absent passage of meconium may be caused by meconium plug syndrome, Hirschsprung disease, meconium ileus (cystic fibrosis), or imperforate anus.
2. Bilious vomiting in the newborn is always abnormal and usually is caused by an intestinal obstruction. Vomiting in the newborn also may be caused by inborn errors of metabolism and congenital adrenal hyperplasia.

E. Urinary problems. Ninety-nine percent of normal full-term infants will urinate by 24 hours. If urination has not occurred within 24 hours, renal ultrasonography should be done and an intravenous fluid challenge may be given.

References, see page 164.

Neonatal Jaundice

Jaundice is defined by a serum bilirubin concentration greater than 5 mg/dL. Clinical jaundice develops in 50% of newborns, and breast-feed infants have an increased incidence of jaundice. Differentiation between physiologic jaundice, which is seen in many infants during the first week of life, and pathologic jaundice is essential because pathologic jaundice is a sign of a more serious condition.

I. Pathophysiology
A. Physiologic versus pathologic jaundice
1. **Physiologic jaundice** is characterized by unconjugated hyperbilirubinemia that peaks by the third or fourth day of life in full-term newborns and then steadily declines by 1 week of age. Asian newborns tend to have higher peak bilirubin concentrations and more prolonged jaundice. Premature infants are more likely to develop jaundice than full-term babies.
2. **Causes of physiologic jaundice**
   a. **Increased bilirubin load** due to the high red blood cell volume in newborns and shortened blood cell survival.
   b. **Deficient hepatic uptake** and deficient conjugation of bilirubin.
   c. **Increased enterohepatic bilirubin** reabsorption.
   d. **Deficient excretion** of bilirubin.
3. **Pathologic jaundice** usually appears within the first 24 hours after birth and is characterized by a rapidly rising serum bilirubin concentration (>5 mg/dL

per day), prolonged jaundice (>7 to 10 days in a full-term infant), or an elevated direct bilirubin concentration (>2 mg/dL). Conjugated hyperbilirubinemia never has a physiologic cause and must always be investigated.

II. Clinical evaluation of jaundice in newborns

A. **History** may reveal abdominal distention, delayed passage of meconium, lethargy, light colored stools, dark urine, low Apgar scores, poor feeding, weight loss, or vomiting.

B. **Physical examination** should seek bruising, cephalhematoma, congenital anomalies, hepatosplenomegaly, pallor, petechiae, or small or large size for gestational age.

C. **Maternal history** should assess history of chorioamnionitis, forceps delivery, vacuum extraction, diabetes, dystocia, or exposure to drugs. Failure to receive immune globulin in a previous pregnancy or abortion that involved risk of isoimmunization should be sought. Family history of jaundice, anemia, liver disease, splenectomy, Greek or Asian race, preeclampsia, or unexplained illness during pregnancy should be assessed.

III. Laboratory evaluation

A. **Diagnostic tests** include blood group typing of both mother and infant, a direct Coombs' test, and measurement of serum bilirubin concentration.

B. **Ill or premature infants**, or those with significant jaundice (serum bilirubin >15 mg/dL) require a complete blood cell count or hemoglobin, reticulocyte count, blood smear, and direct bilirubin level. In infants of Asian or Greek descent, glucose-6-phosphate dehydrogenase (G6PD) should be measured.

IV. Differential diagnosis of unconjugated hyperbilirubinemia

A. **Increased bilirubin production**

1. **Fetal-maternal blood group incompatibility** is one cause of increased bilirubin production. Rh sensitization occurs when an Rh-negative mother is exposed to Rh-positive blood cells. Subsequent Rh-positive fetuses may develop hemolysis. Other minor blood group incompatibilities also can cause hemolysis and jaundice.

2. **ABO incompatibility** is the most common type of isoimmune hemolytic disease. It can occur when the mother's blood group is O and the baby's is A or B. This type of hemolysis is relatively mild.

3. **G6PD deficiency**, a sex-linked disease, is an important cause of hyperbilirubinemia and anemia in infants of Greek and Asian descent.

4. **Abnormalities of the red blood cell membrane**, such as spherocytosis and elliptocytosis, may cause hyperbilirubinemia. Alpha thalassemia may occur in the neonatal period.

5. **Hematoma, occult hemorrhage, or polycythemia** (fetomaternal or twin-to-twin transfusion, delayed cord clamping, intrauterine growth retardation, or maternal diabetes) may lead to hyperbilirubinemia.

B. **Decreased bilirubin excretion**

1. **Delay in intestinal transit time**, because bowel obstruction, increases the enterohepatic circulation. Relief of the obstruction results in a decline in bilirubin concentration.

2. **Crigler-Najjar syndrome** is a rare, inherited, lifelong deficiency of bilirubin excretion. Type I is autosomal recessive. Patients present with extreme jaundice (bilirubin concentration ≥25 mg/dL) and have a very high risk of bilirubin encephalopathy. Type II is autosomal dominant, and it can effectively be treated with phenobarbital.

3. **Neonatal hypothyroidism** is another cause of prolonged indirect hyperbilirubinemia.

C. **Increased bilirubin production and decreased excretion.** Sepsis often causes increased breakdown of red blood cells and decreased hepatic excretion of bilirubin. Certain drugs given to the newborn may also induce hemolysis or decrease bilirubin excretion.

D. **Breast feeding** is associated with neonatal hyperbilirubinemia. In healthy newborns, the danger of an elevated bilirubin concentration is minimal, and switching to formula feeding is unnecessary.

V. **Consequences of unconjugated hyperbilirubinemia. Bilirubin encephalopathy (kernicterus)** is defined as the acute and often fatal syndrome characterized by opisthotonos, hypotonia, a high-pitched cry, and late neurologic sequelae of choreoathetosis, spasticity, upward-gaze paresis, and central hearing loss.

VI. **Treatment**
   A. **Low-risk infants** with minimal jaundice are observed for an increase in the jaundice intensity or a spread to the baby's feet (jaundice advances from head-to-foot).

Management of Hyperbilirubinemia in the Healthy Term Newborn				
	Total serum bilirubin level, mg/dL			
Age (H)	Consider phototherapy	Phototherapy	Exchange transfusion if phototherapy fails	Exchange transfusion and photo-therapy
≤24	...	...	...	...
25-48	≥12	≥15	≥20	≥25
49-72	≥15	≥18	≥25	≥30
>72	≥17	≥20	≥25	≥30

   B. **Phototherapy** with blue light causes photoconversion of bilirubin to a water-soluble product that is excreted in urine and stool. Bilirubin concentrations are measured once or twice a day during phototherapy, and treatment is discontinued when the bilirubin concentration drops below 12 mg/dL.
   C. **Exchange transfusion therapy**. Exchange transfusion is used for emergent treatment of markedly elevated bilirubin and for correction of anemia caused by isoimmune hemolytic disease.

References, see page 164.

Respiratory Disorders of the Newborn

Respiratory distress is a common problem during the first few days of life. Respiratory distress may present with tachypnea, nasal flaring, sternal and intercostal retractions, cyanosis, and apnea.

I. **Transient tachypnea of the newborn**
   A. Transient tachypnea of the newborn (TTN) usually presents as early respiratory distress in term or preterm infants. It is caused by delayed reabsorption of fetal lung fluid.
   B. TTN is a very common, and it is often seen following cesarean section because babies born by cesarean section have delayed reabsorption of fetal lung fluid.
   C. **Symptoms of TTN** include tachypnea, retractions, nasal flaring, grunting, and cyanosis.

    D. **Arterial blood gas** reveals respiratory acidosis and mild-to-moderate hypoxemia.

    E. **Chest x-ray** often reveals fluid in the interlobar fissures and perihilar streaking. Hyperaeration of the lungs and mild cardiomegaly may be seen; alveolar edema may appear as coarse, fluffy densities.

    F. Transient tachypnea of the newborn usually resolves within 12-24 hours. The chest radiograph appears normal in 2-3 days. The symptoms rarely last more than 72 hours.

    G. **Treatment of TTN** consists of oxygen therapy. Infants will usually recover fully, without long-term pulmonary sequelae.

II. **Respiratory distress syndrome**

    A. RDS is a lung disease caused by pulmonary surfactant deficiency. It occurs almost always in preterm infants who are born before the lungs are able to produce adequate amounts of surfactant.

    B. Respiratory distress usually begins at, or soon after, delivery and tends to worsen over time. Infants will have tachypnea, nasal flaring, intercostal and sternal retractions, and expiratory grunting.

    C. **Chest radiography** shows diffuse atelectasis, which appears as reduced lung volume, with homogeneous haziness or the "ground glass" appearance of lung fields, and air bronchograms.

    D. RDS is diagnosed when a premature infant has respiratory distress and a characteristic chest radiograph. The differential diagnosis includes pneumonia caused by group B streptococci.

    E. **Ventilatory management**

       1. Continuous positive airway pressure (CPAP) improves oxygenation and survival (5-7 cm H_2O pressure).

       2. For infants exhibiting respiratory acidosis, hypoxemia or apnea, intermittent positive pressure ventilation will be required in addition to positive end-expiratory pressure (PEEP).

       3. An umbilical or radial arterial line is used to monitor blood gas levels and blood pressure.

    F. **Surfactant replacement therapy**

       1. Surfactant therapy reduces mortality by 30-50% and pneumothorax by 50%.

       2. Surfactant replacement therapy should be initiated as soon as respiratory distress has been clinically diagnosed. As long as the infant requires significant ventilatory support, Survanta (every 6 hours for 4 doses) or Exosurf (every 12 hours for 2 doses) should be given.

    G. **General supportive care.** Sepsis and pneumonia are part of the differential diagnosis of RDS. Presumptive treatment with ampicillin plus gentamicin or cefotaxime usually is given until blood and CSF cultures are negative.

III. **Chronic lung disease (CLD)**

    A. CLD is characterized by hypoxia, hypercarbia, and oxygen dependence that persists beyond 1 month of age. The chest radiograph shows hyperexpansion and focal hyperlucency, alternating with strands of opacification.

    B. CLD is extremely common among infants who have severe RDS treated with mechanical ventilation. The incidence of CLD is inversely proportional to birthweight. Virtually all babies who develop CLD have had mechanical ventilation, suggesting an important role for barotrauma and oxygen toxicity.

    C. Respiratory distress syndrome is the most common pulmonary disease causing CLD. Other neonatal diseases requiring oxygen and mechanical ventilation may also cause CLD, including immature lungs, meconium aspiration syndrome, congenital heart disease, neonatal pneumonia, and aspiration pneumonia.

    D. Signs of CLD include tachypnea and retractions, after extubation. Blood gas measurements show respiratory acidosis with elevated $PaVCO_2$; increased HCO_3 indicates metabolic compensation. Higher inspired oxygen concentration is required to maintain normal oxygenation.

E. Management of CLD consists of minimizing barotrauma. Adjustments in peak pressure should deliver adequate, but not excessive, tidal volume; acceptable minute ventilation can be maintained by monitoring the $PaCO_2$. A moderate degree of respiratory acidosis should be allowed in order to decrease the amount of ventilatory assistance needed, thus reducing the barotrauma. Supplemental oxygen therapy should maintain the PaO_2 in the 60-80 mm Hg range.

F. **Nutrition** is crucial in promoting repair and growth of lung tissue. These infants may need up to 150 kcal/kg/day for optimal growth.

G. **Antibiotics.** Intubated infants who have CLD are susceptible to pneumonia. Close observation for pneumonia and prompt treatment with antibiotics, when pneumonia is suspected, are recommended.

H. **Chest physiotherapy**, with chest percussion, postural drainage and suctioning should be performed as needed.

I. **Diuretic therapy.** Furosemide (1 mg/kg q 24 h IV or PO) may be used. Milder diuretics such as chlorothiazide (10-20 mg/kg per dose q12h PO) and spironolactone (1-2 mg/kg per dose q12h PO) may help reduce airway resistance and improve pulmonary compliance.

J. **Bronchodilators**
   1. Aminophylline (5-7 mg/kg loading dose, followed by 2 mg/kg q6-12h IV) decreases airway resistance and increases lung compliance.
   2. Inhaled albuterol, 0.15 mg/kg q8h, has been shown to benefit pulmonary function.

K. **Corticosteroid Therapy.** Dexamethasone (0.25 mg/kg q12h PO or IV for 3 days, followed by a tapering course over 2-6 weeks) has been shown to improve pulmonary function rapidly and allow earlier extubation.

L. **Home oxygen therapy** should be considered for infants who are receiving supplemental oxygen therapy.

References, see page 164.

Neonatal Resuscitation

Neonatal resuscitation skills are important because of the potential for serious disability or death in high-risk infants and in a few unpredicted full-term, low-risk deliveries.

I. **Preparation**
   A. **Advanced preparation** requires acquisition and maintenance of proper equipment and supplies.
   B. **Immediate preparation**
      1. Suction, oxygen, proper-sized face mask and the resuscitation bag should be checked.
      2. Appropriately sized ET tubes, cut to 13 cm, should be laid out.
      3. Medications should be prepared and an umbilical catheter and tray should be prepared.

Neonatal Resuscitation Equipment and Supplies

Suction Equipment

Bulb syringe
Suction catheters, 5 (or 6), 8, 10 Fr
Meconium aspirator

Mechanical Suction
8 Fr feeding tube and 20 cc syringe

Bag-and-Mask Equipment

Oral airways, newborn and premature sizes
Infant resuscitation bag with a pressure-release valve/pressure gauge to give 90-100% O_2

Oxygen with flow meter and tubing
Cushion rim face masks in newborn and premature sizes

Intubation Equipment

Laryngoscope with straight blades, No. 0 (preterm) and No.1(term newborn).
Extra bulbs and batteries for laryngoscope
Endotracheal tubes, size 2.5, 3.0, 3.5, 4.0 mm

Stylet
Scissors
Gloves

Medications

Epinephrine 1:10,000, 3 cc or 10 cc ampules
Naloxone 0.4 mg/mL,1 mL ampules
Dextrose 10% in water, 250 cc
Sterile water, 30 cc

Volume expanders-one or more of these:
  Albumin 5% solution
  Normal Saline
  Ringer's Lactate solution

Miscellaneous

Radiant warmer and towels or blankets
Stethoscope
Adhesive tape, ½ or 3/4 inch width
Syringes, 1 cc, 3 cc, 5 cc, 10 cc, 20 cc, 50 cc
Umbilical artery catheterization tray
Cardiotachometer and ECG oscilloscope

Alcohol sponges
3-way stopcocks
3 Fr feeding tube
Umbilical tape
Needles, 25, 21, 18 gauge
Umbilical catheters, 3 ½ and 5 Fr

II. Neonatal resuscitation procedures

    A. During delivery, infant evaluation includes assessment of muscle tone, color, and respiratory effort.

    B. After delivery, the infant should be placed on a preheated radiant warmer. The infant should be quickly dried with warm towels. The infant should be placed supine with its neck in a neutral position. A towel neck roll under the shoulders may help prevent neck flexion and airway occlusion.

    C. The **upper airway is cleared** by suctioning; the mouth first, and then the nose, using a bulb syringe. Suctioning should be limited to 5 seconds at a time.

    D. If breathing is effective and pulse is $\geq$100 beats/min, positive pressure ventilation (PPV) is not needed. If cyanosis is present, oxygen should be administered.

E. **Free-flowing oxygen** may be given at a rate of 5 L/min by holding the tubing ½ inch in front of the infant's nose, or an oxygen mask may be used. When the infant's color is pink, the oxygen is gradually discontinued.

F. **Positive pressure ventilation** should be initiated if the infant is not breathing effectively after the initial steps. Tactile stimulation should be administered by gently slapping the soles of the feet or rubbing the back. If the infant is apneic or gasping, begin PPV with 100% O_2. If the heart rate is <100 beats/min, give PPV immediately by bag-mask.

1. **Bag-Mask ventilation**. Ventilations should be given at a rate of 40-60/min. Visible chest wall movement indicates adequate ventilation.

2. **Endotracheal intubation** is initiated if the infant is nonresponsive to bag-mask PPV.

Endotracheal Tube Size and Depth of Insertion From Upper Lip			
Weight	Gestational Age	Size	Depth
<1000 g	<28 weeks	2.5 mm	7 cm
1000-2000 g	28-34 weeks	3.0 mm	8 cm
2000-3000 g	34-38 weeks	3.5 mm	9 cm
3000 g or more	39->40 weeks	4.0 mm	10 cm

G. **Evaluation of heart rate**
1. If the heart rate is ≥100 beats/min, PPV can be gradually discontinued after the infant is breathing effectively.
2. **Chest compressions** should be started if the heart rate is <80 beats/min after 15-30 seconds of adequate ventilation.
   a. Chest compressions are alternated with ventilations at a ratio of 3:1. The combined rate should be 120/min (ie, 80 compressions and 30 ventilations).
   b. After 30 seconds, evaluate the response. If the pulse is ≥80 beats/min, chest compressions can be stopped and PPV continued until the heart rate is 100 beats/min and effective breathing is maintained.
3. **Epinephrine** should be given if the heart rate remains below 80/minute after 30 seconds of PPV and chest compressions.

Neonatal Resuscitation Medications				
Medication	Concentration	Preparation	Dosage	Rate/Precautions
Epinephrine	1:10,000	1 mL	0.1-0.3 mL/kg IV or ET. May repeat in 3-5 min if HR is <80/min	Give rapidly. May dilute 1:1 with normal saline if given via ET
Volume expanders	Whole blood Albumin 5% Normal saline Ringer lactate	40 mL	10 mL/kg IV	Give over 5-10 min by syringe or IV drip
Naloxone	0.4 mg/mL	1 mL	0.1 mg/kg (0.25 mL/kg) IV, ET, IM, SQ	Give rapidly

Medication	Concentration	Preparation	Dosage	Rate/Precautions
Naloxone	1.0 mg/mL	1 mL	1 mg/kg (0.1 mL/kg) IV, ET, IM, SQ	IV, ET preferred. IM, SQ acceptable
Sodium bicarbonate	0.5 mEq/mL (4.2% solution) diluted with sterile water to make 0.5 mEq/mL	20 mL or two 10-mL prefilled syringes	2 mEq/kg IV	Give slowly, over at least 2 min.

4. **Other medications**
   a. **Volume expanders.** Volume expansion is indicated for patients who have known or suspected blood loss and poor response to other resuscitative measures. Albumin 5%, normal saline, or Ringer's lactate can be given in boluses of 10 mL/kg over 5 to 10 minutes.
   b. **Sodium bicarbonate** is recommended during prolonged resuscitation for infants refractory to other measures.
   c. **Naloxone hydrochloride** is given to infants with prolonged respiratory depression following narcotic anesthesia given to the mother within 4 hrs before delivery. Naloxone is contraindicated in infants of mothers who are addicted to narcotics.
5. **Umbilical vessel catheterization** is recommended when vascular access is required. The large, centrally located, thin-walled and flat vein is used, and a 3.5 or 5.0 Fr radiopaque catheter is inserted into the vein until a free flow of blood can be aspirated.

References, see page 164.

General Pediatrics

Diabetes Mellitus

Diabetes mellitus consists of hyperglycemia caused by insulin deficiency, impairment of insulin action, or both. Five percent of the population is affected by diabetes, 10% of whom have type 1 diabetes.

I. **Classification of diabetes mellitus**
   A. Diabetes mellitus is classified into two types: type 1 and type 2.
   B. **Type 1 diabetes**
      1. Type 1 diabetes is caused by absolute insulin deficiency. Most cases among children and adolescents (95%) result from autoimmune destruction of the beta cells of the pancreas.
      2. The peak age at diagnosis is 12 years, and 75-80% of individuals develop type 1 diabetes before age 30.
   C. **Type 2 diabetes** is caused by insulin resistance and relative insulin deficiency. Most type 2 diabetics do not require insulin injections and are obese.

Criteria for Diagnosis of Diabetes

Fasting plasma glucose 126 mg/dL or higher
or
Random plasma glucose 200 mg/dL or higher with symptoms of diabetes (fatigue, weight loss, polyuria, polyphagia, polydipsia)
or
Abnormal two-hour 75-g oral glucose tolerance test result, with glucose 200 mg/dL or higher at two hours
Any abnormal test result must be repeated on a subsequent occasion to establish the diagnosis

---

II. **Management of diabetic ketoacidosis**
   A. DKA can be seen at the time of diagnosis of type 1 diabetes or in the patient who has established disease if diabetes management is inadequate. DKA is caused by insulin deficiency, which leads to hyperglycemia and ketogenesis.
   B. **Symptoms** include polyuria, polydipsia, hyperpnea with shortness of breath, vomiting, and abdominal pain. Hyperosmolar dehydration and acid/base and electrolyte disturbances occur.
   C. **Rehydration**
      1. **Immediate evaluation** should assess the degree of dehydration by determining capillary refill, skin temperature, and postural heart rate and blood pressure.
      2. Initial fluid resuscitation consists of a 10-mL/kg bolus of 0.9% saline over 30-60 minutes, repeated if hypovolemic shock persists. Patients then should begin to receive maintenance fluid requirements added to the calculated fluid deficit (>2 y: 30 mL/kg for mild deficit, 60 mL/kg for moderate deficit, 90 mL/kg for severe deficit; <2 y: 50 mL/kg for mild deficit, 100 mL/kg for moderate deficit, 150 mL/kg for severe deficit). The sodium concentration of the fluid should provide 50% of the sodium deficit in the first 12 hours and the remainder in the next 36 hours (75 to 125 mEq/L sodium chloride).

Laboratory Monitoring During DKA	
Blood glucose:	At presentation, then hourly by fingerstick with glucose meter
Serum sodium and potassium:	At presentation, then at 4- to 6-h intervals
Acid/base status:	At presentation, then at 2- to 4-h intervals. Venous pH and serum carbon dioxide
Serum urea nitrogen, complete blood count, acetone and cultures can be obtained at presentation.	

D. **Potassium replacement.** DKA is associated with total body potassium depletion. This deficit should be replaced by infusing potassium chloride at a rate of 3 mEq/kg per 24 hours after completion of the normal saline fluid resuscitation. If the patient requires more than 4 mEq/kg of a potassium infusion, 50% can be administered as potassium phosphate to help prevent hyperchloremic acidosis and hypophosphatemia.

E. **Lowering the glucose level**
   1. Regular insulin should be initiated as an intravenous infusion of 0.1 U/kg per hour. The goal of therapy is to lower the glucose level by 50 to 100 mg/dL per hour.
   2. Once the glucose level is in the range of 250 to 350 mg/dL, 5% glucose should be initiated; when the glucose level is between 180 to 240 mg/dL, the infusate can be changed to 10% glucose.

F. **Correcting acidosis.** Alkali therapy is usually not necessary to correct the acidosis associated with DKA. If acidosis is severe, with a pH less than 7.1, sodium bicarbonate can be infused slowly at a rate of 1 to 3 mEq/kg per 12 hours and discontinued when the pH exceeds 7.2.

III. **Long-term diabetes management**
   A. Intensive management of diabetes results in a significant reduction in the development of diabetic complications: a 76% reduction in retinopathy, a 39% reduction in microalbuminuria, and a 60% reduction in neuropathy.

Target Blood Glucose Range (Preprandial)	
Age	**Glucose Levels (mg/dL)**
Infants, toddlers	120-220
Preschool children	100-200
School-age children	70-150

B. **Insulin regimens**
   1. **Starting dose of insulin.** Most newly diagnosed patients with type 1 diabetes can be started on 0.2 to 0.4 units of insulin per kg. Adolescents often need more. The dose can be adjusted upward every few days based upon symptoms and blood glucose measurements.

2. **Dosing regimens.** Insulin should be provided in two ways – as a basal supplement with an intermediate- to long-acting preparation and as pre-meal bolus doses of short-acting insulin (to cover the extra requirements after food is absorbed).
3. **Monomeric insulins**
   a. **Insulin lispro (Humalog)** has an onset of action within 5 to 15 minutes, peak action at 30 to 90 minutes, and a duration of action of 2 to 4 hours. Insulin lispro is the preferred insulin preparation for pre-meal bolus doses.
   b. **Insulin aspart (Novolog)** is another monomeric insulin. It is a rapid-acting insulin analog with an onset of action within 10 to 20 minutes. Aspart reaches peak concentrations in 40-50 minutes and has a duration of action of 3-5 hours. Insulin aspart, like insulin lispro, can be injected immediately before meals, and has a shorter duration of action than regular insulin. Insulin aspart has a slightly slower onset and longer duration of action than insulin lispro.

Pharmacokinetics of Insulin Preparations				
Type of insulin	Onset of action	Peak of action	Duration of action	Common pitfalls
Insulin lispro (Humalog)	5 to 15 minutes	45 to 75 minutes	2 to 4 hours	Hypoglycemia occurs if the lag time is too long; with high-fat meals, the dose should be adjusted downward.
Insulin aspart (Novolog)	10 to 20 minutes	40 to 50 minutes	3 to 5 hours	
Regular insulin (Humulin R)	30 minutes	2 to 4 hours	5 to 8 hours	The insulin should be given 20 to 30 minutes before the patient eats.
Insulin glargine (Lantus)	1 to 3 hours	5 to 7 hours	13 to 18 hours	Has a constant glucose-lowering profile without peaks and valleys, allowing it to be administered once every 24 hours.
NPH insulin (Humulin N)	1 to 3 hours	6 to 12 hours	18 to 28 hours	In many patients, breakfast injection does not last until the evening meal; administration with the evening meal does not meet insulin needs on awakening.
Lente insulin (Humulin L)	1 to 3 hours	4 to 8 hours	13 to 20 hours	Loses its effect if it is left in the syringe for more than a few minutes.

Total Daily Insulin Dosage		
<5 Years (U/kg)	**5-11 Years (U/kg)**	**12-18 Years (U/kg)**
0.6-0.8	0.75-0.9	0.8-1.5
Newly diagnosed patients and those who are in the remission phase may require less insulin.		

4. **Twice-daily regimens**. If the goal is relief from hyperglycemic symptoms with a regimen that is simple, then twice-daily NPH insulin will be effective in many patients. Injection of regular plus NPH insulin before breakfast and before dinner results in four peaks of insulin action, covering the morning, afternoon, evening, and overnight, but the peaks tend to merge.

5. **Insulin glargine (Lantus)**. While NPH insulin is the insulin most commonly given at bedtime, insulin glargine may be equally effective for reducing HbA1c values and cause less hypoglycemia.

C. **Insulin regimens for intensive therapy of diabetes mellitus**

1. **Multiple daily injections**. The most commonly used multiple-dose regimen consists of twice-daily injections of regular and intermediate-acting insulin (NPH).

2. Although a twice-daily regimen improves glycemic control in most patients, the morning dose of intermediate-acting insulin may not be sufficient to prevent a post-lunchtime rise in blood glucose concentrations. The intermediate-acting insulin administered before the evening meal may not be sufficient to induce normoglycemia the next morning unless a larger dose is given, which increases the risk of hypoglycemia during the night. If necessary, the twice-daily regimen can be converted into a three- or four-injection program.

3. In contrast to NPH insulin, the time-action profile for insulin glargine has virtually no peak, which may make it the ideal basal insulin for intensive insulin therapy in type 1 diabetes.

4. **Monomeric insulins**, insulin lispro and insulin aspart, may be most useful in patients in whom high postprandial blood glucose concentrations and unexpected high blood glucose values at other times are problems.

5. Inhaled insulin may become an alternative to monomeric insulins in the future. It causes a very rapid rise in serum insulin concentrations (similar to that achieved with subcutaneous insulin lispro). Typical premeal doses consists of 1.5 units per kg taken five minutes before a meal.

D. **Blood glucose monitoring.** Children and adolescents should test their blood glucose levels at least four times a day, before meals and at bedtime. Quarterly measurement of hemoglobin A1c (HbA1c) assesses glycemic control and reflects the average blood glucose over the last 120 days.

Assessment of HbA1c Values	
HbA1c Values	**Level of Glycemic Control**
HbA1c >10%	Poor or minimal
HbA1c 8.0-10.0%	Average

HbA1c Values	Level of Glycemic Control
<8.0%	Excellent or intensive

References, see page 164.

Menstrual Disorders

The median age of menarche is 12.8 years, and the normal menstrual cycle is 21 to 35 days in length. Bleeding normally lasts for 3 to 7 days and consists of 30 to 40 mL of blood. Cycles are abnormal if they are longer than 8 to 10 days or if more than 80 mL of blood loss occurs. Soaking more than 25 pads or 30 tampons during a menstrual period is abnormal.

I. Pathophysiology
  A. **Regular ovulatory menstrual cycles** often do not develop until 1 to 1.5 years after menarche, and 55-82% of cycles are anovulatory for the first 2 years after menarche. Anovulatory cycles typically cause heavier and longer bleeding.
  B. **Adolescents** frequently experience irregular menstrual bleeding patterns, which can include several consecutive months of amenorrhea.
II. Amenorrhea
  A. **Primary amenorrhea** is defined as the absence of menarche by age 16. Puberty is considered delayed and warrants evaluation if breast development (the initial sign of puberty in girls) does not begin by the age of 13. The mean time between the onset of breast development and menarche is 2 years. Absence of menses within 2 to 2.5 years of the onset of puberty should be evaluated.
  B. **Secondary amenorrhea** is defined as the absence of 3 consecutive menstrual cycles or 6 months of amenorrhea in patients who have already established regular menstrual periods.

Differential Diagnosis of Amenorrhea

Pregnancy
Hormonal Contraception
Hypothalamic-related Disorders
    Chronic or systemic illness
    Stress
    Athletics
    Eating disorders
    Obesity
    Drugs
    Tumor
Pituitary-related Disorders
    Hypopituitarism
    Tumor
    Infiltration
    Infarction
Ovarian-related Disorders
    Dysgenesis
    Agenesis
    Ovarian failure
    Resistant ovary

Outflow Tract-related Disorders
    Imperforate hymen
    Transverse vaginal septum
    Agenesis of the vagina, cervix, uterus
    Uterine synechiae
Androgen Excess
    Polycystic ovarian syndrome
    Adrenal tumor
    Adrenal hyperplasia (classic and nonclassic)
    Ovarian tumor
Other Endocrine Disorders
    Thyroid disease
    Cushing syndrome

C. Amenorrhea with pubertal delay

1. **Hypergonadotropic hypogonadism** is caused by ovarian failure associated with elevated gonadotropin levels. An elevated FSH will establish this diagnosis.

   a. **Turner syndrome (XO)** may cause ovarian failure and a lack of pubertal development. Females with Turner syndrome have streak gonads, absence of one of the X chromosomes, and inadequate levels of estradiol. They do not initiate puberty or uterine development. This syndrome is characterized by short stature, webbed neck, widely spaced nipples, shield chest, high arched palate, congenital heart disease, renal anomalies, and autoimmune disorders (thyroiditis, Addison disease). It may not be diagnosed until adolescence, when pubertal delay and amenorrhea occur together.

   b. **Ovarian failure** resulting from autoimmune disorders or exposure to radiation or chemotherapy may also cause amenorrhea with pubertal delay associated with hypergonadotropic hypogonadism.

2. **Hypogonadotropic hypogonadism** is caused by hypothalamic dysfunction or pituitary failure. Low or normal levels of LH and FSH will be present, and decreased estradiol levels may be present.

   a. **Abnormalities of the pituitary and hypothalamus**, and other endocrinopathies (thyroid disease and Cushing syndrome) may present with pubertal delay and low gonadotropin levels.

      (1) Amenorrhea may be caused by problems at the level of the pituitary gland, such as congenital hypopituitarism, tumor (pituitary adenoma), or infiltration (hemochromatosis).

      (2) **Prolactin-secreting pituitary adenoma (prolactinoma)** is the most common pituitary tumor. Prolactinomas present with galactorrhea, headache, visual fields cuts, and amenorrhea. Elevated prolactin levels are characteristic.

      (3) **Craniopharyngioma** is another tumor of the sella turcica that affects hypothalamic-pituitary function, presenting with pubertal delay and amenorrhea.

      (4) Other disorders associated with galactorrhea and amenorrhea include hypothyroidism, breast stimulation, stress associated with trauma or surgery, phenothiazines, and opiates.

   b. **Hypothalamic suppression** is most commonly caused by stress, competitive athletics, and dieting (anorexia nervosa).

   c. **Hypothalamic abnormalities** associated with pubertal delay include Laurence-Moon-Biedl, Prader-Willi, and Kallmann syndromes. Laurence-Moon-Biedl and Prader-Willi present with obesity. Kallmann syndrome is associated with anosmia.

D. Amenorrhea with normal pubertal development

1. **Pregnancy** should be excluded when amenorrhea occurs in a pubertally mature female.

2. **Contraceptive-related amenorrhea** occurs with depot medroxyprogesterone (Depo-Provera); it does not require intervention; however, a pregnancy test should be completed.

3. **Uterine synechiae (Asherman syndrome)** should be suspected in amenorrheic females with a history of abortion, dilation and curettage, or endometritis.

4. **Sheehan syndrome (pituitary infarction)** is suggested by a history of intrapartum bleeding and hypotension.

5. **Other disorders associated with amenorrhea and normal pubertal development.** Ovarian failure, acquired abnormalities of the pituitary gland (prolactinoma), thyroid disease, and stress, athletics, and eating disorders may cause amenorrhea after normal pubertal development. Polycystic ovarian disease, which is usually associated with irregular bleeding, can also present with amenorrhea.

E. **Genital tract abnormalities**
   1. **Imperforate hymen** will appear as a membrane covering the vaginal opening. A history of cyclic abdominal pain is common, and a midline abdominal mass may be palpable.
   2. **Transverse vaginal septum** may cause obstruction. It is diagnosed by speculum examination.
   3. **Agenesis of the vagina** appears as a blind-ended pouch. Normal pubertal development of breast and pubic hair occurs, but menarche does not occur.
   4. **Androgen insensitivity (testicular feminization syndrome)** is another common cause of vaginal agenesis.
      a. Breast development and a growth spurt occur, but little if any pubic or axillary hair is present. These women have an XY chromosomal pattern with intra-abdominal or inguinal testes that produce testosterone, but an X-linked inherited defect of the androgen receptor prevents response to testosterone.
      b. Female-appearing external genitalia are present, but the uterus and vagina are absent. During puberty, breast development occurs because of conversion of androgens to estrogens.
      c. The testes are at increased risk for developing tumors and must be removed. Hormone replacement therapy is provided to initiate puberty.

F. **Polycystic ovary syndrome**
   1. PCO is the most common cause of persistent irregular menses. Only 70% of patients have polycystic ovaries on ultrasound. The most common symptom is irregular periods beginning with menarche; however, intervals of amenorrhea may also occur. Signs include hirsutism, acne, clitoromegaly, and obesity (50%). Insulin resistance, glucose intolerance, and lipid abnormalities are common.
   2. Increased facial hair and midline hair over the sternum and lower abdomen are often present. If hirsutism is severe, an ovarian and adrenal tumor or adrenal enzyme deficiency should be excluded.
   3. PCO is probably an autosomal recessive disorder that affects ovarian steroidogenesis. Ovulation occasionally can occur spontaneously; therefore, amenorrhea secondary to pregnancy must be considered.

G. **Clinical evaluation of amenorrhea**
   1. **Chronic or systemic illness**, eating disorders, and drug use, including hormonal contraception, should be excluded. Tanner staging, pelvic examination, and possibly pelvic ultrasonography should be completed.
   2. **Absence of the uterus**, vagina, or both requires a chromosomal analysis, which can determine if the karyotype is XX or XY, and it can help differentiate between müllerian agenesis and androgen insensitivity.
   3. If the anatomy is normal, **LH, FSH, and estradiol** are indicated in order to distinguish ovarian failure from hypothalamic dysfunction. High FSH and LH levels and a low estradiol level are indicators of gonadal dysgenesis (Turner syndrome) or autoimmune oophoritis. Normal or low LH, FSH, and estradiol levels indicate hypothalamic suppression, central nervous system tumor, or an endocrinopathy (eg, hypothyroidism).
   4. **Pregnancy** must always be excluded if the individual is mature pubertally.
   5. **Free-T4, TSH, and prolactin** levels are checked to exclude hypothyroidism and hyperprolactinemia. If the prolactin level is elevated, an MRI is necessary to exclude prolactinoma.
   6. **Hirsutism and acne** are indicative of androgen excess and PCO. Total testosterone and dehydroepiandrosterone sulfate (DHEAS) levels are necessary to exclude ovarian and adrenal tumors. A testosterone level >200 ng/dL and DHEAS >700 µg/dL require further investigation to exclude a tumor.

7. **A morning 17-hydroxyprogesterone level** will screen for nonclassic adrenal hyperplasia. A 17-hydroxyprogesterone >2 ng/mL is followed by an ACTH stimulation test to diagnose 21-hydroxylase deficiency.

8. An elevated LH-to-FSH ratio is common with PCO; an ultrasonographic examination may detect polycystic ovaries.

H. Treatment of amenorrhea

1. **Anovulation** and the resulting lack of progesterone increases the risk of endometrial hyperplasia and endometrial cancer. Oral medroxyprogesterone or an oral contraceptive (OCs) should be prescribed to eliminate this risk. Oral progestins can be given cyclically for 12 days every month or every third month.

2. **PCO** is treated with OCs to regulate menses and to decrease androgen levels. Electrolysis and spironolactone (50 mg tid) can decrease hirsutism.

3. **Hypoestrogenic and anovulatory patients** with hypothalamic suppression caused by anorexia, stress, or strenuous athletics should modify their behavior and be prescribed calcium and hormonal replacement therapy (OCs) to reduce the risks of osteoporosis.

4. **Turner syndrome or ovarian failure** requires estrogen and progesterone at a dosage sufficient to induce pubertal development, after which time they can be switched to an OC.

III. Abnormal vaginal bleeding

A. Abnormal vaginal bleeding is characterized by excessive uterine bleeding or a prolonged number of days of bleeding. The most common cause of abnormal vaginal bleeding in adolescence is anovulation. Abnormal bleeding is common during the first 1 to 2 years after menarche because anovulatory cycles are frequent.

B. Differential diagnosis of abnormal vaginal bleeding

1. **Pregnancy**, pregnancy-related complications, sexually transmitted diseases, pelvic inflammatory disease, and retained tampons should be excluded.

2. **Vaginal tumors**, uterine or cervical carcinoma, and uterine myomas are rare in adolescents.

3. **Blood dyscrasias or coagulation defects** may occasionally be the initial presentation of abnormal vaginal bleeding.

4. **Hormonal contraceptives** are a common cause of breakthrough bleeding.

C. Clinical evaluation of irregular vaginal bleeding

1. Age of menarche, menstrual pattern, amount of bleeding, symptoms of hypovolemia, history of sexual activity, genital trauma, and symptoms of endocrine abnormalities or systemic illness should be evaluated.

2. Postural vital signs may suggest hypovolemia. A pelvic examination should assess pelvic anatomy and exclude trauma, infection, foreign body, or a pregnancy-related complication. Pelvic ultrasonography can be used to further assess pelvic anatomy.

Differential Diagnosis of Abnormal Vaginal Bleeding

Pregnancy-related. Ectopic pregnancy, abortion

Hormonal contraception. Oral contraceptives, depo-medroxyprogesterone

Hypothalamic-related. Chronic or systemic illness, stress, athletics, eating disorder, obesity, drugs

Pituitary-related. Prolactinoma, craniopharyngioma

Outflow tract-related. Trauma, foreign body, vaginal tumor, cervical carcinoma, polyp, uterine myoma, uterine carcinoma, intrauterine device

Androgen excess. Polycystic ovarian syndrome, adrenal tumor, ovarian tumor, adrenal hyperplasia

Other endocrine causes. Thyroid disease, adrenal disease

Hematologic causes. Thrombocytopenia, clotting abnormalities, abnormalities of platelet function, anticoagulant medications

Infectious causes. Pelvic inflammatory disease, cervicitis

---

   3. Laboratory evaluation
      a. **A pregnancy test and complete blood count** should be completed.
      b. **A history of a very heavy period with menarche** or repeated prolonged or heavy menses warrants a prothrombin time and partial thromboplastin time to screen for bleeding abnormalities; a bleeding time and von Willebrand screening panel will identify more specific coagulation disorders.
      c. **Signs of androgen excess** indicate a need to exclude PCO.
      d. **Chronic irregular vaginal bleeding** mandates that prolactinoma and endocrine abnormalities (thyroid disease) be excluded.
   D. Treatment of irregular vaginal bleeding
      1. **Mild bleeding or shortened cycles** associated with a normal physical examination and normal vital signs requires only reassurance.
      2. **Mild anemia** associated with stable vital signs is treated with a 35 to 50 mcg monophasic combination OC as follows: One pill QID x 4 days. One pill TID x 3 days. One pill BID x 7 days. One pill QD x 7-14 days. Stop all pills for 7 days and then begin cycling on a low dose OCP QD.
      3. The patient should be continued on low-dose OCs for 3 to 4 months before allowing resumption of normal cycles. Iron therapy should be included.
      4. **If the hematocrit is <7-8 mg/dL or if vital signs are unstable,** hospitalization is recommended. Intravenous conjugated estrogens (Premarin), 25 mg IV every 4-6 hours for 24 hours, will stop the bleeding quickly. Conjugated estrogen therapy is followed immediately by OCs and iron therapy. Blood transfusion is warranted only if the patient is severely symptomatic. Dilatation and curettage is used as a last resort; however, it is rarely necessary.
      5. **Antiprostaglandin medications (NSAIDs)** decrease menstrual blood loss significantly by promoting platelet aggregation and vasoconstriction. They do not have the hormonal side effects of OCs, and they can be used alone in mild cases of abnormal vaginal bleeding.
IV. Dysmenorrhea
   A. Fifty percent of adolescents experience dysmenorrhea
   B. **Primary dysmenorrhea** consists of crampy lower abdominal and pelvic pain during menses that is not associated with pelvic pathology. It is the most common form of dysmenorrhea, usually beginning 6 months to 1 year after menarche.
   C. **Secondary dysmenorrhea** is defined as painful menses associated with pelvic pathology (bicornate uterus, endometriosis, PID, uterine fibroids and polyps, cervical stenosis, ovarian neoplasms). If dysmenorrhea is severe, obstructing lesions of the genital tract should be excluded. Endometriosis is the most common cause (50%) of chronic pelvic pain in adolescents.

D. **Evaluation of dysmenorrhea**
1. **Gynecologic history** should determine the relationship of the pain to the menstrual cycle, severity, and sexual activity.
2. **If the pain is mild**, easily relieved by NSAIDs, and the physical examination (including the hymen) are normal, a speculum examination is not necessary.
3. **Severe pain** requires a pelvic examination to exclude genital tract obstruction, adnexal and/or uterosacral pain (endometriosis), PID, or a mass. Ultrasonography is useful for evaluating pelvic abnormalities or obstruction.

E. **Treatment of dysmenorrhea**
1. **Initial treatment** consists of a prostaglandin synthesis inhibitor, initiated with the onset of bleeding and continued for as long as pain lasts. Gastric irritation can be reduced by taking the drug with food.
   a. **Mefenamic acid (Ponstel)** 500 mg loading dose, then 250 mg q6h.
   b. **Ibuprofen (Advil)** 400-600 mg q4-6h.
   c. **Naproxen sodium (Aleve)** 550 mg load, then 275 mg q6h.
   d. **Naproxen (Naprosyn)** 500 mg load, then 250 mg q6-8h.
2. **Oral contraceptives** are also very effective and can be added if the antiprostaglandin is not fully effective.

References, see page 164.

Nocturnal Enuresis

Nocturnal enuresis affects approximately 5 to 7 million children in the United States. Parents may become concerned about nocturnal enuresis when their child reaches 5 to 6 years of age. There is a slight male predominance of 60% for nocturnal enuresis. Etiologic factors include genetics, sleep arousal dysfunction, urodynamics, nocturnal polyuria, psychological components, and maturational delay.

I. **Clinical evaluation**
A. **History**
1. A detailed toilet training history and a family history of enuresis should be sought. Other pertinent details include the onset and pattern of wetting, voiding behavior, sleep pattern, parasomnias, medical conditions, daytime urinary symptoms, bowel habits, and psychosocial factors.
2. Urgency or a history of small, frequent voids suggests bladder instability or small bladder capacity. Dysuria suggest a urinary tract infection. Polyuria and polydipsia suggest diabetes insipidus or mellitus. Encopresis suggests constipation. Nighttime snoring suggests adenoidal hypertrophy.

B. **Physical examination**
1. Most children who have nocturnal enuresis will have normal findings on physical examination. Height, weight, and blood pressure should be recorded.
2. A palpable bladder, palpable stool, ectopic ureter, signs of sexual abuse, or abnormal gait should be sought. Cremasteric, anal, abdominal, and deep tendon reflexes that reflect spinal cord function all should be tested.
3. The skin of the lower back should be inspected for a sacral dimple, hair patches, or vascular birthmarks, which indicate spinal dysraphism. Mouth breathing may suggest sleep apnea with associated enuresis due to adenoidal hypertrophy.
4. Direct observation of the urinary stream is important if findings suggest an abnormality. Bladder capacity can be measured in the office by having the child drink 12 oz of fluid on arrival, then voiding into a calibrated cup.

C. **Laboratory/imaging studies.** All children should have urinalysis of a clean-catch midstream urine specimen. The ability to concentrate urine to 1.015 or greater rules out diabetes insipidus and the absence of glucose rules out diabetes mellitus. A urine culture should be obtained if the child has dysuria or an abnormal urinalysis.

II. Treatment

A. Nonpharmacologic therapy

1. **Motivational therapy.** The child should be taken out of diapers or training pants and encouraged to empty the bladder completely prior to going to bed. The child should participate in morning cleanup. Fluids should be restricted for 2 hours prior to bedtime.

2. **Behavioral therapy**

   a. **Hypnotherapy** involves having the child practice imagery of awakening to urinate in the toilet or staying dry all night.

   b. **Dry-bed training** involves waking the child over several nights, and having the child walk to the toilet when voiding is needed. The eventual goal is to have the child self-awaken to void.

   c. **Enuresis alarms** have the highest overall cure rate. Alarm systems can be used in combination with behavioral therapy or pharmacotherapy. The cure rate may be as high as 70% long-term.

B. Pharmacotherapy. Medication for nocturnal enuresis seldom should be considered before 8 years of age.

1. **Imipramine (Tofranil)**

   a. Imipramine increases bladder capacity and also may decrease detrusor muscle contractions. The starting dose is 25 mg taken 1 hour before bedtime for children ages 6 to 8 years and 50 to 75 mg for older children and adolescents. The dose may be increased in 25-mg increments weekly up to 75 mg. Therapy may continue from 3 to 9 months, with a slow tapering over 3 to 4 weeks. Imipramine is inexpensive. The success rate is 15 to 50%.

   b. Mild side effects include irritability, dry mouth, decreased appetite, headaches, and sleep disturbances. Overdose can be lethal.

2. **DDAVP (Stimate)**

   a. DDAVP is a synthetic analog of arginine vasopressin (ADH). It decreases urine volume. The bioavailability is only 1% for the tablet and 10% for the nasal spray. The initial dose of DDAVP is 20 mcg PO or one 10-mcg puff in each nostril within 2 hours of bedtime. The dose may be increased in increments of 10 mcg every 1 or 2 weeks up to a maximum dose of 40 mcg. Patients may remain on medication for 3 to 6 months, then should begin a slow decrease of the dose by 10 mcg/mo. If oral medication is preferred, the starting dose is 0.2 mg (one tablet) 1 hour before bedtime. If there is no response within 1 week, the dose can be titrated by 0.2 mg up to a maximum of 0.6 mg nightly.

   b. Side effects of DDAVP are rare and include abdominal discomfort, nausea, headache, and epistaxis. Symptomatic hyponatremia with seizures is very rare. Contraindications include habit polydipsia, hypertension, and heart disease. About 22% become dry with DDAVP.

   c. DDAVP's high initial response rate is attractive for episodic use for summer camp and sleepovers.

C. Age-related treatments

1. **Younger than age 8 years.** Motivational and behavioral methods that assist the child in waking to void and that praise successful dryness are recommended.

2. **Ages 8 through 11 years.** The enuresis alarm gives the best results in terms of response rate and low relapse rate. Intermittent use of medication such as DDAVP can be useful for special events.

3. **Ages 12 years and older.** If use of an enuresis alarm does not stop wetting episodes, continuous use of medication is justified.

References, see page 164.

Poisoning

Poisoning is defined as exposure to an agent that can cause organ dysfunction, leading to injury or death. Children less than 6 years of age account for 60.8% of poisonings.

I. Clinical evaluation of poisoning
   A. **The type of toxin** involved should be determined. The time of the exposure and how much time has elapsed should be assessed.
   B. **The dose of the toxin** should be assumed to be the maximum amount consistent with the circumstances of the poisoning.
   C. **Munchausen syndrome by proxy**
      1. Chemical child abuse should be suspected when childhood poisonings are associated with an insidious and/or inexplicable presentation (eg, recurrent acidosis, polymicrobial sepsis, recurrent malabsorption syndrome, factitious hypoglycemia, failure to thrive).
      2. The syndrome is referred to as "Munchausen syndrome by proxy" when the abuse is perpetrated by a caretaker. Agents may include aspirin, codeine, ethylene glycol, fecal material, insulin, ipecac, laxatives, phenothiazines, table salt, and vitamin A.

II. Physical examination
   A. The first priority in a severely poisoned child is to maintain an airway, ventilation, and circulation.
   B. The vital signs, breath odors, skin, gastrointestinal, cardiovascular, respiratory, and neurologic systems should be assessed.

Physical Findings Associated with Specific Drugs and Chemicals	
Symptom or Sign	**Agents**
Fever	Amphetamines, anticholinergics, antihistamines, aspirin, cocaine, iron, phencyclidine, phenothiazines, thyroid, tricyclic antidepressants
Hypothermia	Barbiturates, carbamazepine, ethanol, isopropanol, narcotics, phenothiazines
Breath odors: 　Mothballs 　Fruity 　Garlic 　Bitter almond 　Peanuts	 Naphthalene, paradichlorobenzene Isopropanol, acetone, nail polish remover Arsenic, organophosphates Cyanide N-3-pyridylmethyl-N-4-nitrophenylurea (VACOR rat poison)
Hypertension	Amphetamines, cocaine, ephedrine, ergotism, norepinephrine, phenylpropanolamine, tricyclic antidepressants (early)
Hypotension	Antihypertensives, arsenic, barbiturates, benzodiazepines, beta blockers, calcium channel blockers, carbon monoxide, cyanide, disulfiram, iron, nitrites, opiates, phenothiazines, tricyclic antidepressants (late)

Physical Findings Associated with Specific Drugs and Chemicals	
Symptom or Sign	**Agents**
Tachypnea	Amphetamine, cocaine, carbon monoxide, cyanide, iron, nicotine, phencyclidine, salicylates
Hypoventilation	Alcohols, anesthetics, barbiturates, benzodiazepines, botulism, chlorinated hydrocarbons, cholinesterase-inhibiting pesticides, cyclic antidepressants, narcotics, nicotine, paralytic shellfish poisoning, solvents, strychnine
Coma	Alcohols, anticonvulsants, barbiturates, benzodiazepines, carbon monoxide, chloral hydrate, cyanide, cyclic antidepressants, hydrocarbons, hypoglycemics, insulin, lithium, narcotics, phenothiazines, salicylates, sedative-hypnotics, solvents
Seizures	Amphetamines, camphor, carbon monoxide, cocaine, gyromitra mushrooms, isoniazid, lead, lindane, nicotine, pesticides, phencyclidine, salicylates, strychnine, theophylline, tricyclic antidepressants
Miosis	Narcotics, organophosphates, phenothiazines, phencyclidine
Mydriasis	Amphetamine, anticholinergics, antihistamines, atropine, cocaine, phenylpropanolamine, tricyclic antidepressants
Nystagmus	Phencyclidine, phenytoin
Peripheral neuropathy	Acrylamide, carbon disulfide, heavy metals

C. Skin examination
1. Cyanosis suggests hypoxia secondary to aspiration (eg, hydrocarbon) or asphyxia (eg, apnea due to central nervous system depressants).
2. The adolescent substance abuser may have needle tracks along veins or scars from subcutaneous injections. Urticaria suggests an allergic reaction. Jaundice may signify hemolysis from naphthalene mothballs.

D. Cardiovascular effects
1. Sympathetic stimulation can cause hypertension with tachycardia.
2. Hypotension is caused by beta adrenergic blockade, calcium channel blockade, sympatholytic agents, cellular toxins, psychopharmaceutical agents, disulfiram-ethanol, and shock associated with iron or arsenic.

E. Respiratory effects
1. **Tachypnea and hyperpnea** may result from salicylate poisoning. Nervous system stimulants may be associated with tachypnea. Cellular poisons will increase the respiratory rate.
2. **Central nervous system depressants** may depress the respiratory drive.
3. **Apnea** may be associated with toxins causing weakness of respiratory muscles. The respiratory examination may reveal poisoning-associated wheezing (eg, beta-blocker overdose or inhalants) or crackles (aspiration pneumonia, pulmonary edema).

F. Neurologic examination
1. **Depressed consciousness**, confusion, delirium, or coma may result from

toxins, such as ethanol. Central nervous system stimulants or neurotransmitter antagonists produce seizures.

   2. **Pupils.** Dilated pupils can be caused by sympathetic stimulation (eg, amphetamine, cocaine). Constricted pupils are caused by parasympathetic stimulation (eg, organophosphate pesticides) or sympathetic blockade (eg, phenothiazines).
   3. **Sensorimotor examination** may reveal peripheral anesthesia caused solvents, pesticides, or acrylamide.
   4. **Neurologic signs of substance abuse**
       a. **Ethanol, isopropyl alcohol, ethylene glycol, or methanol** can cause an alcoholic state of intoxication. Amphetamine or cocaine often cause agitation, euphoria, or paranoia. Lysergic acid diethylamide (LSD), mescaline or amphetamines can cause visual or auditory hallucinations.
       b. **Benzodiazepines and narcotics** (oxycodone) can cause drowsiness, slurred speech, confusion, or coma. Phencyclidine (PCP) causes agitation, dissociative delusional thinking, rhabdomyolysis, and rotatory nystagmus. Glue or gasoline sniffing can result in exhilaration, grandiose delusions, irrational behavior, and sudden death from cardiac dysrhythmias.

III. **Laboratory assessment**
   A. **Toxic screens**
       1. The history and physical examination will usually provide enough information to make a diagnosis and begin therapy. Occasionally, toxin screening of blood and/or urine can confirm the diagnosis.
       2. A toxic screen of the blood and urine may include assays for acetone, acetaminophen, amphetamines, anticonvulsants, antidepressants, antihistamines, benzodiazepines, ethanol, isopropanol, methanol, narcotics, neuroleptics, or phencyclidine.
   B. **Serum osmolarity**
       1. **The osmolar gap** is derived from the measured serum osmolality minus the calculated serum osmolality ($2 \times Na + BUN/2.8 + glucose/18$). When exogenous osmoles are present (eg, ethanol, isopropyl alcohol, methanol, acetone, or ethylene glycol), the osmolar gap will be elevated.
       2. **Anion gap acidosis**
           a. Lactic acid (eg, in ethanol, isoniazid, iron poisonings), ketoacids (eg, diabetes, ethanol), or exogenous organic acids may cause a metabolic acidosis.
           b. Metabolic acidoses are classified as either increased anion gap ($[Na+ K] - [Cl + HCO_3]$) above 15 mEq/L (ethylene glycol, iron, isoniazid, methanol, or salicylate), or depressed anion gap (lithium), or normal anion gap (laxatives, colchicine).
   C. **Other frequently ordered tests**
       1. **Hepatic and renal function** should be monitored because most toxins are detoxified in the liver and/or excreted in the urine. Many poisonings are accompanied by rhabdomyolysis (elevated creatinine phosphokinase levels) from seizures, hyperthermia, or muscle spasms.
       2. **Urine that fluoresces under Wood lamp** examination is diagnostic of antifreeze poisoning.
       3. **Chest and abdominal radiographs** may show radiopacities from calcium tablets, chloral hydrate, foreign bodies, iodine tablets, phenothiazine and antidepressant tablets, and enteric-coated capsules.
       4. **Serial electrocardiograms** are essential with antiarrhythmic drugs, beta-blockers, calcium channel blockers, lithium, phenothiazines, theophylline, or tricyclic antidepressants.

IV. Diagnostic trials
    A. For a few poisons, a "diagnostic trial" of an antidote can implicate an agent as the cause of a poisoning.

Diagnostic Trials			
Toxin	**Diagnostic Trial**	**Route**	**Positive Response**
Benzodiaz-epine	Flumazenil 0.02 mg/kg	IV	Consciousness improves
Digitalis	Specific Fab antibodies	IV	Dysrhythmia resolves, hyperkalemia improves, consciousness improves
Insulin	Glucose 1 g/kg	IV	Consciousness improves
Iron	Deferoxamine 40 mg/kg	IM	Pink "vin rose" urine
Isoniazid	Pyridoxine 5 g	IV	Seizures abate
Opiate	Naloxone 0.1 mg/kg	IV	Consciousness improves
Phenothiazine	Diphenhydramine 1 mg/kg	IV	Dystonia and torticollis resolve

V. Management
    A. Poison centers can help with the diagnosis and management of poisonings, and assist in locating exotic antidotes.

    B. Initial management of poisoning involves maintaining an airway, providing ventilatory support, securing vascular access, and initiating resuscitation.

    C. Decontamination

        1. **Skin, mucous membrane, or eye exposures** should be washed with a stream of lukewarm water for 15 to 20 minutes. Soap is used to decontaminate skin exposures.

        2. **Gastric lavage**

            a. **Decontamination** by lavage is preferred over emesis in the emergency department because it is controllable. Contraindications include nontoxic ingestions, ingestions in which the substance is already past the stomach or absorbed, and caustic or hydrocarbon ingestions. It is most successful when performed within 90 minutes of the ingestion. For toxins associated with delayed gastric emptying (eg, aspirin, iron, antidepressants, antipsychotics) or for those that can form concretions (eg, iron, salicylates), lavage may be beneficial hours later.

            b. **A large-bore (24-32F) orogastric tube** is used, and 100- to 200-cc aliquots of warm, normal saline are infused/withdrawn until no more pill fragments are detectable in the lavage fluid or until about 2 liters have been exchanged.

            c. **Activated charcoal** is effective for absorbing most drugs, but it is ineffective for alcohols, caustics, cyanide, heavy metals, lithium, and some pesticides.

            d. Overdoses of carbamazepine, tricyclic antidepressants, and procainamide are managed with multiple doses of charcoal. Contraindications to charcoal include a poisoning where esophageal endoscopy is contemplated, one in which the toxin is not adsorbed by charcoal, or a poisoning in which the patient has an ileus, gastrointestinal hemorrhage, or repeated retching.

3. Enhanced elimination

a. Multiple doses of charcoal also can enhance elimination by "gastrointestinal dialysis." Repetitive doses of charcoal are recommended for phenobarbital, salicylate, and theophylline poisoning.

b. A cathartic, such as magnesium citrate, is recommended when charcoal is used because charcoal is constipating. Hemodialysis or hemoperfusion can be life-saving for severe intoxications.

VI. Specific toxins

A. Acetaminophen (APAP)

1. Single overdoses of greater than 150 mg/kg can cause liver failure. Nausea and abdominal pain are common. The patient may vomit repeatedly, be mildly lethargic, or remain asymptomatic. At 24 to 36 hours after the ingestion, abdominal tenderness and rising serum transaminase levels signify onset of hepatitis that peaks in severity by 96 hours.

2. The Rumack nomogram predicts the likelihood of hepatitis. The peak concentration is measured 4 hours after the ingestion; levels greater than 200 mcg/mL at 4 hours are associated with liver toxicity.

3. When acetaminophen has been taken in high dose, or when acetaminophen levels are in the range likely to cause hepatotoxicity, N-acetylcysteine (NAC) is given at a loading dose of 140 mg/kg, followed by 17 doses of 70 mg/kg separated by 4-hour intervals.

4. Once NAC has been started because of one toxic level, the full course should be given; there is no need to get repeated APAP concentrations.

B. Alcohols

1. Alcohols include ethanol, ethylene glycol, methanol, and isopropyl alcohol. Antifreeze contains ethylene glycol, Sterno and windshield wiper fluid contain methanol, jewelry cleaners and rubbing alcohol contain isopropanol.

2. All of the alcohols cause inebriation, loss of motor control and coma. Ethylene glycol may cause acidosis, renal failure, and seizures. Methanol may cause metabolic acidosis, seizures, and blindness. Isopropyl alcohol can produce gastritis, ketosis, and hypotension.

3. Concentrations of ethylene glycol or methanol >20 mg/dL require the use of ethanol therapy to block alcohol dehydrogenase conversion to the toxic metabolites; hemodialysis is indicated for concentrations >50 mg/dL. Isopropanol or ethanol intoxications usually require only close monitoring with frequent measurements of serum glucose. Respiratory depression, seizures, and coma from ethanol poisoning and levels >300-400 mg/dL require hemodialysis.

C. Caustics

1. **Drain cleaners** contain sodium hydroxide or sulfuric acid; toilet cleaners may contain hydrochloric or sulfuric acids.

2. **Laundry or dishwasher detergents** may contain sodium metasilicate or sodium triphosphate.

3. **Signs of caustic ingestion** include lip or tongue swelling; burning pain; dysphagia; drooling; and whitish or red plaques on the tongue, buccal or palatal mucosa, or in the perioral area. Caustics can cause severe burns to the esophagus or stomach even in the absence of symptoms.

4. **Inhalations** are managed with humidified oxygen. Skin exposures are washed carefully with soap and water and then treated like any other burn.

5. **Strongly alkaline agents** damage the upper esophagus. **Hydrochloric, sulfuric (muriatic), and other acids** damage the lower esophagus and stomach.

6. **Treatment of caustic ingestions.** The child should be given nothing by mouth, and endoscopic evaluation should be performed 12 to 24 hours after the ingestion. Emesis, lavage and charcoal are contraindicated.

D. Foreign body ingestion

1. **Aspirated objects** will cause symptoms of choking, gasping, coughing, cyanosis, wheezing, fever, and poor air entry. While chest radiography can confirm the diagnosis, a negative film does not rule out aspiration. A foreign body requires immediate removal by bronchoscopy.

2. **Ingestion of disc batteries** requires removal when lodged in the esophagus; those in the stomach or beyond should be followed with repeated abdominal films every 2 to 3 days to ensure passage. Disc batteries that have remained in one position for more than 7 days may require surgical removal. Coins or other foreign bodies past the esophagus can be managed with serial radiographs and parental vigilance for their passage.

E. Hydrocarbons

1. **Aliphatic hydrocarbons** include kerosene, mineral oil, gasoline, and petrolatum. Kerosene and gasoline are capable of causing an aspiration pneumonia and CNS depression. Petrolatum, mineral oil and motor oil do not carry significant risk of injury. Aliphatic hydrocarbons in small doses are not harmful if left in the stomach. Emesis is contraindicated because of the risk of aspiration; decontamination should be attempted only if a very large dose was taken.

2. **Aromatic hydrocarbons,** such as xylene or toluene, are toxic. Aromatic hydrocarbon ingestions necessitate lavage.

3. **Aspiration pneumonia** is suggested by gasping, choking, coughing, chest pain, dyspnea, cyanosis, leukocytosis, and fever. A chest radiograph may not be diagnostic until hours after ingestion.

F. Iron

1. Iron is present in many children's multivitamins, although the worst cases of iron poisoning usually involve prenatal vitamins, which contain 60 mg of elemental iron per tablet. Iron is a metabolic poison and is corrosive to gastric mucosa, resulting in shock.

2. Ferrous sulfate is 20% elemental iron, ferrous fumarate 33%, and ferrous gluconate 11%. Little toxicity is seen at a dose of elemental iron less than 20 mg/kg. Mild symptoms of poisoning are seen at doses of 20-60 mg/kg; moderate-to-severe symptoms at doses of 60 to 100 mg/kg; life-threatening symptoms at doses greater than 100 mg/kg; and a lethal dose is 180 to 300 mg/kg.

3. **Early symptoms** include nausea, vomiting, fever, hemorrhagic diarrhea, tachycardia, hypotension, hyperglycemia, and acidosis. Intermediate symptoms (8 to 48 hours after ingestion) may include obtundation, coma, fulminant hepatitis, hypoglycemia, clotting abnormalities, pulmonary edema, and renal tubular dysfunction.

4. **Laboratory findings** include a metabolic acidosis with a high anion gap, an abdominal radiograph showing radiopaque pills in the stomach, an elevated white blood cell count greater than 15,000/mm^3, and an elevated blood glucose >150 mg/dL. A serum iron concentration, obtained 4 hours after the ingestion, of less than 300 mcg/dL is not toxic; 300 to 500 mcg/dL is mildly toxic; 500 to 1000 mcg/dL is moderately to severely toxic; greater than 1000 mcg/dL is life-threatening.

5. **Treatment.** Decontamination by lavage should be initiated; charcoal is not effective. Volume expansion with intravenous fluids, correction of electrolyte/acid-base disturbances, and intravenous deferoxamine are recommended.

G. Salicylates

1. Aspirin overdoses greater than 150 mg/kg are toxic. Salicylates are locally corrosive, and tablets can form bezoars near the gastric outlet. Salicylates stimulate the central respiratory center, so that the metabolic acidosis is compensated

by a respiratory alkalosis.

2. **Early symptoms** of toxicity include gastrointestinal pain, nausea, vomiting, tinnitus, confusion, lethargy, and fever. Respirations often are rapid and deep. Severe poisonings can be associated with seizures, coma, and respiratory and cardiovascular failure.

3. **Laboratory findings** include hypocalcemia, hypomagnesemia, hypokalemia, and hyperglycemia (early) or hypoglycemia (late).

4. **Serum aspirin concentration** obtained 2 and 6 hours after the ingestion higher than 30 mg/dL are considered toxic, those greater than 70 mg/dL are associated with severe symptoms, and those greater than 100 mg/dL are life-threatening.

5. **Management** includes lavage, which may be effective as long as 4 to 6 hours after the ingestion. Multiple-dose activated charcoal is effective. Correction of acidemia, hypokalemia, and hypocalcemia are important. Hemodialysis is indicated for serum concentrations greater than 100 mg/dL.

References, see page 164.

Developmental Pediatrics

Infant Growth and Development

Infancy consists of the period from birth to about two years of age. Advances occur in physical growth, motor development, cognitive development, and psychosocial development.

I. **Physical growth milestones**
   A. Birth weight is regained by 2 weeks of age and doubles by 5 months. During the first few months of life, this rapid growth continues, after which the growth rate decelerates.

Average Physical Growth Parameters				
Age	Head circumference	Height	Weight	Dentition
Birth	35.0 cm (13.8 in) +2 cm/mo (0 to 3 mo) +1 cm/mo (3 to 6 mo) +0.5 cm/mo (6 to 12 mo) Mean = 1 cm/mo	50.8 cm (20.0 in)	3.0 to 3.5 kg (6.6 to 7.7 lb) Regains birthweight by 2 wk Doubles birthweight by 5 mo	Central incisors--6 mo Lateral incisors--8 mo
1 year	47.0 cm (18.5 in)	76.2 cm (30.0 in)	10.0 kg (22 lb) Triples birthweight	First molars--14 mo Canines--19 mo
2 years	49.0 cm (19.3 in)	88.9 cm (35.0 in)	12.0 to 12.5 kg (26.4 to 27.5 lb) Quadruples birthweight	Second molars--24 mo

   B. **Occipitofrontal circumference**
      1. **Microcephaly** is associated with an increased incidence of mental retardation, but there is no direct relationship between small head size and decreased intelligence. Microcephaly associated with genetic or acquired disorders usually has cognitive implications.
      2. **Macrocephaly** may be caused by hydrocephalus, which is associated with learning disabilities. Macrocephaly without hydrocephalus is associated with cognitive deficits caused by metabolic or anatomic abnormalities. Fifty percent of cases of macrocephaly are familial and have no effect on intellect. When evaluating the infant with macrocephaly, the finding of a large head size in one or both parents is reassuring.
   C. **Height and weight**
      1. Although the majority of individuals who are of below- or above-average size are otherwise normal, there is an increased prevalence of developmental disabilities

in these two groups.

2. Many genetic syndromes are associated with short stature; large stature syndromes are less common. When considering deviation from the norm, short stature in the family is reassuring.

D. Dysmorphism. Most isolated minor dysmorphic features are inconsequential; however, the presence of three or more indicative of developmental dysfunction. Seventy-five percent of minor superficial dysmorphisms can be found by examining the face, skin, and hands.

II. Motor development milestones

A. Motor milestones are ascertained from the developmental history and observation. Gross motor development begins with holding head up, rolling and progresses to sitting, and then standing, and ambulating.

B. Fine motor development

1. In the first year of life, the pincer grasp develops. During the second year of life, the infant learns to use objects as tools during play.

2. Reaching becomes more accurate, and objects are initially brought to the mouth for oral exploration. As the pincer grasp and macular vision improve, precise manual exploration replaces oral exploration.

C. Red flags in motor development

1. Persistent listing to one side at 3 months of age often is the earliest indication of neuromotor dysfunction.

2. Spontaneous frog-legs posturing suggests hypotonia/weakness, and scissoring suggests spastic hypertonus. Early rolling (1 to 2 months), pulling directly to a stand at 4 months (instead of to a sit), W-sitting, bunny hopping, and persistent toe walking may indicate spasticity.

3. Hand dominance prior to 18 months of age should prompt the clinician to examine the contralateral upper extremity for weakness associated with a hemiparesis.

III. Cognitive development milestones

A. Language is the single best indicator of intellectual potential; problem-solving skills are the next best measure. Gross motor skills correlate least with cognitive potential; most infants with mental retardation walk on time.

B. Problem-solving skills

1. The 1-year-old child recognizes objects and associates them with their functions. Thus, he begins to use them functionally as "tools" instead of mouthing, banging, and throwing them.

2. Midway through the second year, the child begins to label objects and actions and categorize them, allowing the child to match objects that are the same and later to match an object to its picture.

3. **Object permanence**

   a. Prior to the infant's mastery of object permanence, a person or object that is "out of sight" is "out of mind," and its disappearance does not evoke a reaction.

   b. The child will progress to finding an object that has been hidden under a cloth.

   c. The next skill in this sequence is the ability to locate an object under double layers (eg, a cube is placed under a cup and then the cup is covered with a cloth).

4. **Causality.** Initially, the infant accidentally discovers that his actions produce a certain effect. The infant then learns that actions cause consistent effects.

C. Language development

1. Receptive language skills reflect the ability to understand language. Expressive language skills reflect the ability to make thoughts, ideas, and desires known to others.

2. **Prespeech period (0 to 10 months).** Receptive language is characterized by an increasing ability to localize sounds, such as a bell. Expressive language consists of cooing. At 3 months, the infant will begin vocalizing after hearing an adult speak. At 6 months of age, the infant adds consonants to the vowel sounds in a repetitive fashion (babbling). When a random vocalization (eg, "dada") is interpreted by the parents as a real word, the parent will show pleasure and joy. In so doing, parents reinforce the repeated use of these sounds.

3. **Naming period (10 to 18 months).** The infant's realizes that people have names and objects have labels. The infant begins to use the words "dada" and "mama" appropriately. Infants next recognize and understand their own names and the meaning of "no." By 12 months of age, some infants understand as many as 100 words. They can follow a simple command as long as the speaker uses a gesture. Early in the second year, a gesture no longer is needed.

4. The infant will say at least one "real" word (ie, other than mama, dada) before his first birthday. At this time, the infant also will begin to verbalize with sentence-like intonation and rhythm (immature jargoning). As expressive vocabulary increases, real words are added (mature jargoning). By 18 months, the infant will use about 25 words.

5. **Word combination period (18 to 24 months).** Children begin to combine words 6 to 8 months after they say their first word. Early word combinations are "telegraphic" (eg, "Go out"). A stranger should be able to understand at least 50% of the infant's speech.

D. **Red flags in cognitive development**
1. Language development provides an estimate of verbal intelligence; problem-solving provides an estimate of nonverbal intelligence. If deficiencies are global (ie, skills are delayed in both domains), there is a possibility of mental retardation.

2. When a discrepancy exists between problem-solving and language abilities, with only language being deficient, the possibility of a hearing impairment or a communication disorder should be excluded. If either language or problem-solving skills is deficient, the child is at high risk for a learning disability later.

3. All children who have delayed language development should receive audiologic testing to rule out hearing loss. Deaf infants will begin to babble on time at 6 months, but these vocalizations will gradually decline thereafter.

IV. **Psychosocial development**
A. **Emotional development.** Emotions are present in infancy and motivate expression (pain elicits crying).

B. **Social development**
1. Social milestones begin with bonding, which reflects the feeling of the caregiver for the child. Attachment represents the feeling of the infant for the caregiver, and it develops within a few months.

2. When recognition of and attachment to a caregiver develops, the simple sight of this person will elicit a smile. The infant becomes more discriminating in producing a smile as he begins to differentiate between familiar and unfamiliar faces. The infant learns to use smiling to manipulate the environment and satisfy personal needs.

3. Temperament represents the style of a child's emotional and behavioral response to situations.

C. **Adaptive skill development.** Adaptive skills consist of the skills required for independence in feeding, dressing, toileting, and other activities of daily living. Development of adaptive skill is influenced by the infant's social environment, and by motor and cognitive skill attainment.

D. **Red flags in psychosocial development**
1. **Colic** may be an early indication of a "difficult" temperament.

2. **Delay in the appearance of a smile** suggests an attachment problem, which may be associated with maternal depression. In severe cases, child neglect or abuse may be suspected.
3. **Failure to develop social relationships** suggests autism when it is accompanied by delayed or deviant language development and stereotypic behaviors.
4. **Delays in adaptive skills** may indicate overprotective parents or an excessive emphasis on orderliness.

References, see page 164.

Toddler Development

Toddlerhood consists of the years from about 1 to 3 years of age. Affective development is highlighted by the toddler's striving for autonomy and independence, attachment to family, and the development of impulse control. Cognitive development is characterized by the transition from sensorimotor to preoperational thought.

I. **Growth rate and physical appearance**
   A. After the rapid growth of infancy, the rate of growth slows in the toddler years. After age 2, toddlers gain about 5 lb in weight and 2.5 inches in height each year. Growth often occurs in spurts. Between the ages of 2 and 2.5 years, the child will have reached 50% of his adult height.
   B. Growth of the lower extremities often is accompanied by tibial torsion and physiologic bowing of the legs, which usually corrects by age 3 years. The percentage of body fat steadily decreases from 22% at age 1 year to about 15% at age 5 years.

II. **Gross motor skills**
   A. Most children walk without assistance by 18 months. At 2 years, the stiff, wide-leg gait of early toddlerhood becomes a flexible, steady walking pattern, with heel-toe progression.

Gross Motor Abilities
18 Months
• Walking fast, seldom falling • Running stiffly • Walking up stairs with one hand held • Seating self in a small chair • Climbing into an adult chair • Hurling a ball
24 Months
• Running well without falling •   Walking up and down stairs alone • Kicking a large ball
36 Months
• Walking up stairs by alternating feet • Walking well on toes • Pedaling a tricycle • Jumping from a step • Hopping two or three times

III. Fine motor skills

A. The 18-month-old can make a tower of four blocks. One year later, he can stack eight blocks. Most 18-month-olds will hold the crayon in a fist and scribble spontaneously on paper.

Fine Motor Abilities
18 Months
• Making a tower of four cubes • Releasing 10 cubes into a cup • Scribbling spontaneously • Imitating a vertically drawn line
24 Months
• Building a seven cube tower • Aligning two or more cubes to form a train • Imitating a horizontally drawn line • Beginning circular strokes • Inserting a square block into a square hole
36 Months
• Copying a circle • Copying bridges with cubes • Building a tower of 9 to 10 blocks • Drawing a person's head

IV. Affective development

A. **Autonomy and independence.** Because of improved motor skills, the transition from infancy to toddlerhood is marked increased autonomy and independence. The toddler may refuse to eat unless allowed to feed himself, and the child may no longer may be willing to try new foods.

B. **Impulse control.** Toddlers begin to develop impulse control. The 18-month-old may have minimal impulse control and display several temper tantrums each day. Most 3-year-olds have some degree of self-control.

C. **Successful toileting** usually occurs toward the end of the third year when the child becomes able to control his sphincter, undress, get onto the potty, and has the willingness to participate. Success with consistent daytime dryness usually is not achieved until about 2.5 to 3 years of age.

Social/Emotional Skills
18 Months
• Removing a garment • Feeding self and spilling food • Hugging a doll • Pulling a toy

24 Months
• Using a spoon; spilling little food • Verbalizing toileting needs • Pulling on a simple garment • Verbalizing immediate experiences • Referring to self by name

36 Months
• Showing concern about the actions of others • Playing cooperatively in small groups • Developing the beginnings of true friendships • Playing with imaginary friends

    D. Attachment refers to the bond that forms between the infant and the caregiver. Disorders of attachment may result from inconsistent caregiving and are more common in the presence of poverty, drug use, or emotional illness.

    E. Temperament determines how a child approaches a given situation. Ten percent of children are less adaptable and tend to be emotionally negative and are considered "difficult."

V. Cognitive development

    A. Toddlerhood is characterized by a transition from sensorimotor to preoperational thinking. Preoperational thought is marked by the development of symbolic thinking, as the child becomes capable of forming mental images and begins to solve problems. Progression from sensorimotor to symbolic thought occurs typically between 18 and 24 months of age.

    B. Complete object permanence has developed, and the child can find an object under a blanket, despite not seeing it hidden.

    C. By 3 years, he can draw primitive figures that represent people, and he develops elaborate play and imagination.

Intellectual Abilities

18 Months
• Pointing to named body parts • Understanding of object permanence • Beginning to understand cause and effect

24 Months
• Forming mental images of objects • Solving problems by trial and error • Understanding simple time concepts

36 Months
• Asking "why" questions • Understanding daily routine • Appreciating special events, such as birthdays • Remembering and reciting nursery rhymes • Repeating three digits

VI. Language

A. Beginning around age 2 years, toddlers use language to convey their thoughts and needs (eg, hunger). The 18-month-old has a vocabulary of at least 20 words, consisting primarily of the names of caregivers, favorite foods, and activities.

B. After 18 months, the toddler begins to put together phrases. Early two and three word sentences are referred to as "telegraphic speech," and about 50% of what the child says should be intelligible to strangers.

C. By the age of 3 years, the vocabulary increases to about 500 words, and 75% of speech is understandable to strangers. He begins to make complete sentences, and frequently asks "why" questions.

Language Skills

18 Months

- Looking selectively at a book
- Using 10 to 20 words
- Naming and pointing to one picture card
- Naming an object (eg, ball)
- Following two-directional commands

24 Months

- Using two to three word sentences
- Using "I," "me," "you"
- Naming three picture cards
- Naming two objects
- Knowing four-directional commands

36 Months

- Using four to five word sentences
- Telling stories
- Using plurals
- Recognizing and naming most common objects

References, see page 164.

Preschooler Development

I. Family relationships

A. **Separation**. The average 3-year-old child can separate easily from parents. Some children cope by adopting a transitional object, usually a soft object, which serves as a symbolic reminder of the parent.

B. **Fears and fantasies**. Early fantasy, may be indistinguishable from reality, resulting in a tendency for fears. By the age of 4, children frequently have frightening dreams that they can state are "not real."

C. **Temper tantrums** are characteristic of 2-year-olds, but they should be infrequent by age 5, although there is another peak at 6 years in response to the stresses of schooling.

D. **Oppositionality**. Preschool children comply with adult requests about 50% of the time. Parents who are authoritative and firm but also warm, encouraging, and rational are more likely to have children who are self-reliant and self-controlled.

A system of discipline should include positive reinforcement for desired behaviors; consequences for undesired behaviors; and interactions that promote the parent-child relationship.

E. Sibling interactions
   1. Factors associated with greater sibling rivalry, include opposite gender, difficult temperament, insecure pattern of attachment, family discord, and corporal punishment. Preschool children often "regress" when a new baby is born, exhibiting increased naughtiness, thumb sucking, and altered toileting.
   2. Sibling classes, avoidance of forced interactions, a strong relationship between the older child and the father, good support for the mother, individual time with each parent, and talking about the new baby are helpful.

II. Peer relationships
   A. Play
      1. At the age of 2 years, most play is parallel. By the age of 3, children should have mastered aggression and should be able to initiate play with a peer, have joint goals in their play together, and take turns. Fantasy or pretend play gains prominence at about age 3.
      2. Pretend friends are very common in children up to the age of 4. Mastery of aggressive impulses should improve after 2½ years of age.

Peer Relationships				
	2-year visit	3-year visit	4-year visit	5-year visit
Amount of interaction	Parallel play with peers, copies others, self-talk, solitary play, offers toy, plays games	Takes on a role, prefers some friends over others, plays associatively with others	Interactive games, best friend <2 y difference, may visit neighbor by self, plays cooperatively with others	Group of friends
Duration of interaction	Briefly alone from adult, sudden shifts in intensity of activity	20 min with peers	Prefers peer play to solitary	
Level of fantasy	Symbolic doll, action figures; mimics domestic activities	Simple fantasy play; unfamiliar may be monsters	Elaborate fantasy play, distinguishes fantasy from reality, tells fanciful tales	Make-believe and dress up
Imaginary friends		May have one	Common	If present, private
Favorite toys/activities	Things that move, turn, or fit together; water; books; music; listens to stories	Listens to stories, dresses and undresses dolls	Sings a song, dances, acts, listens to stories	

	2-year visit	3-year visit	4-year visit	5-year visit
Rule use	Able to take turns, beginning property rights, "mine," "right places"	Shares some	Shares spontaneously, follows rules in simple games, facility with rules, alternately demanding/cooperative	Follows rules of the game, follows community rules
Aggression	Aggressive to get things	Negotiates conflicts	Wants to please friends	

Development of Independence

	2-year visit	3-year visit	4-year visit	5-year visit
Eating	Uses utensils	Spills little, pours some	Helps set table	Helps cook
Dressing	Undresses, pulls on simple garment	Dresses with supervision, unbuttons some	Dresses all but tying	
Toileting	Clean and dry, but with adult effort and motivation	Clean and dry by self-motivated approach	Independent	

Motor and Cognitive Play Skills

	2-year visit	3-year visit	4-year visit	5-year visit
Pencil grip	Point down	Awkward, high		Standard
Drawings Identifies Imitates Copies Person-body parts	Vertical, scribble	Shapes Horizontal, cross Circle before cross 2 parts	Longer line Cross before square 6 parts	Directions Square before triangle 10, including head, body, arms, legs
Scissors	One hand	Across paper	Cuts out square	
Block tower	6-9	Tower of 10		
Block figure	Aligns 4 for train	3 block bridge	5 block gate	Steps

	2-year visit	3-year visit	4-year visit	5-year visit
Other	Turns pages 1 at a time			Ties knot in string, prints letters

III. Communication

A. The 2-year-old has a vocabulary of approximately 150 to 500 words. The child should be speaking in two-word utterances (eg, "my Mommy" or "more milk"). They often mimic what others say (echolalia) up to age 2.5 years. Criterion for referral at 2 years of age is a less than a 50-word vocabulary or not putting two words together.

B. The 3-year-old speaks in simple sentences of three or four words. Sentence length increases by one or two words annually throughout the preschool period, with at least the same number of words that the child is old. The typical 3-year-old can count three items, and a 4-year-old can count four items. A 4-year-old who cannot converse with familiar people with sentences averaging three words should be evaluated.

C. A 5-year-old should use complete sentences containing five words. The 5-year-old can count ten objects or more and should understand "before," "after," and "until"; "if, then." They can discuss emotions and tell jokes. Preschool children who have expressive language disorders tend to speak less often and convey less information than their peers.

D. Strangers should be able to understand 25% to 50% of what the 2-year-old child says. By 3 years of age, strangers should be able to understand the child 75% of the time. By the age of 4, strangers can understand the child 100% of the time, although errors in "r," "s," "l," "sh," and "th" sounds are not uncommon until age 7.

E. Dysfluency (aberration of speech rate and rhythm) occurs transiently between about 2.5 and 4 years of age. Persistent and worsening stuttering beyond the age of 4 should be evaluated.

Communication Skills in Preschoolers

	2-year visit	3-year visit	4-year visit	5-year visit
Vocabulary	No jargon; 150 to 500 words			Definitions
Sentence length	2 words	3 to 4 words	4 to 5 words	
Intelligibility to stranger	25%	75%	100%	
Grammatic forms	Verbs, some adjectives and adverbs	Plurals, pronouns	Past tense	Future tense

	2-year visit	3-year visit	4-year visit	5-year visit
Typical examples	Talks about current action, no jargon, names pictures	Tells own age and sex, counts to 3	Describes recent experiences, can sing songs, gives first and last names, counts to 4, identifies gender	Counts to 10 or more, recognizes letters of the alphabet, knows telephone number and address
Fluency	Dysfluency common	Dysfluency common	Some dysfluency	Dysfluencies not expected

Comprehension

	2-year visit	3-year visit	4-year visit	5-year visit
Number step command	100% for 1 without gesture	2	3	
Number of body parts	Names 1, identifies 7			
Number of colors		2 named	4 named	
Gender		Self	Self and others	
Own names	Refers to self by name	First and last		
Numbers counted	Says "2" (not counted)	Counts to 3		10, knows number
Relationships		Which is bigger, under	Which is longer, 2 opposites	

Motor development

	2-year visit	3-year visit	4-year visit	5-year visit
Walks forward	Slightly bent	Swings arms	Tandem walks	
Walks backward	10 ft			Tandem
Runs	Changing direction	Alternating arms		
Climbs	Out of crib (2.5 y)	High equipment		

	2-year visit	3-year visit	4-year visit	5-year visit
Jumps	Both feet off floor	26 to 30 in from both feet	32 in, one foot leads	Over 10 in
Jumps down	Step with both feet	16 in, lands on one foot first	18 in, lands on both feet	
Stairs-up	One step at a time	Without rail, alternating		
Stairs-down	One step at a time	Alternating, no rail	Alternating	
Stands on one foot	Tries	1 sec on 1 foot	5 to 6 sec on each foot	10 sec
Kicks	kicks ball 6 ft			
Hops		3 hops in place	5 forward	20 ft forward 10 times
Throws	Throws 5 ft	Bounce, overhand	10 ft, 1 or 2 arms	
Catches		Straight arms	Bent arm	Bounce pass
Skips				Skips
Pedals		10 ft, tricycle		

References, see page 164.

School-age Child Development

Middle childhood consists of years six through twelve. This period is characterized by the ability to consider several factors, evaluate oneself and perceive the opinions of others. Self-esteem is essential to the development of the school-aged child. Healthy development requires increasing separation from parents and the ability to find acceptance in the peer group and to meet challenges outside the home.

I. Physical development

   A. Growth during the period averages 3-3.5 kg (7 lb) and 6 cm (2.5 in) per year. Growth occurs in irregular spurts lasting on average 8 wk, three to six times per year. The head grows only 2-3 cm in circumference.

   B. Loss of deciduous (baby) teeth begins at about age 6 years of age.

   C. Muscular strength, coordination, and stamina increase progressively, as does the ability to perform complex movements such as dancing, shooting basketballs, or playing the piano.

   D. The sexual organs remain physically immature, but interest in gender differences and sexual behavior remains of interest to many children. Masturbation is common.

II. Cognitive and language development

A. School-aged children increasingly apply rules, consider multiple points of view, and interpret their perceptions in view of realistic principles.

B. By third grade, children need to be able to sustain attention through a 45-min period. The first 2 years of elementary school are devoted to acquiring the fundamentals of reading, writing, and basic mathematics. By third or fourth grade, children use those fundamentals to learn increasingly complex materials.

C. Factors that determine classroom performance include eagerness to please adults, cooperativeness, competitiveness, willingness to work for a delayed reward, self-confidence, and ability to risk trying.

D. Beginning in third or fourth grade, children increasingly enjoy strategy games and word play (puns and insults) that exercise growing cognitive and linguistic mastery.

Perceptual, Cognitive, and Language Processes Required for Elementary School Success		
Process	**Description**	**Associated Problems**
Perceptual		
Visual analysis	Ability to break a complex figure into components and understand their spatial relationships	Persistent letter confusion (eg, between b, d, and g); difficulty with basic reading and writing
Proprioception and motor control	Ability to sense body position by feel and unconsciously program complex movements	Poor handwriting, requiring excessive effort
Phonologic processing	Ability to perceive differences between similar sounding words and to break down words into sounds	Delayed receptive language skills; attention and behavior problems caused by not understanding direction
Cognitive		
Long-term memory	Ability to acquire "automatic" skills	Delayed mastery of the alphabet (reading and writing letters); slow handwriting; inability to progress beyond basic mathematics
Selective attention	Ability to listen and ignore distractions	Difficulty following multistep instructions, completing assignments, and behaving well
Sequencing	Ability to remember things in order; ability to understand time	Difficulty organizing assignments, planning, spelling, and telling time

Language		
Receptive language	Ability to comprehend complex constructions, function words (eg, if, when, only, except), nuances of speech, and long blocks of language (e.g., paragraphs)	Difficulty following directions; wandering attention; problems with reading comprehension; problems with peer relationships
Expressive language	Ability to recall required words effortlessly (word finding), to control meanings by varying position and word endings, to construct meaningful paragraphs and stories	Difficulty expressing feelings and using words for self- defense, with resulting frustration and physical acting out; struggling during "circle time" and with language skills.

I. **Social and emotional development**
   A. School-aged children identify with same-sex parents, adopting them as role models. The parents' moral judgments are internalized as the superego. School-aged children display decreased emotional lability toward parents and an increasing involvement in relationships outside of the home.
   B. Social and emotional development proceeds in three contexts: the home, the school, and the neighborhood. The home is the most influential. Milestones of a school child's increasing independence include the first sleepover at a friend's house and the first time at overnight camp.
   C. Parents should make demands for effort in school and extracurricular activities, celebrate successes, and offer unconditional acceptance when failures occur. Regular chores provide an opportunity for children to contribute to the family, supporting self-esteem.
   D. Siblings have critical roles as competitors, loyal supporters, and role models. Sibling relationships influence self-image, approach to conflict resolution and interests.
   E. The beginning of school coincides with a child's further separation from the family and the increasing importance of teacher and peer relationships. In addition to friendships that may persist for months or years, experience with a large number of superficial friendships and antagonisms contributes to a child's growing social competence. Popularity, an important part of self-esteem, may be won through possessions (having the right toys) as well as through personal attractiveness, accomplishments, and social skills.
   F. Conformity is rewarded in school-aged children. Some children conform readily and enjoy easy social success; those who adopt individualistic styles or have visible differences may be stigmatized.
   G. Dangers such as busy streets, bullies, and strangers tax school-aged children's common sense and resourcefulness. Interactions with peers call on increasing conflict resolution or pugilistic skills. Children may feel powerlessness in the world, and compensatory fantasies of being powerful may lead to a fascination with superheroes.

References, see page 164.

Attention-deficit/Hyperactivity Disorders

Attention-deficit/hyperactivity disorder (AD/HD) affects about 5% of girls and 10% of boys of elementary age. AD/HD can interfere with an individual's ability to inhibit behavior (impulsivity) and/or function efficiently in goal-oriented activities (inattention). Symptoms of AD/HD emerge in early childhood and continue to be present into adulthood in up to 70% of cases.

I. **Clinical evaluation**
   A. Three behavioral subtypes of ADHDs are defined: predominantly inattentive, predominantly hyperactive/impulsive, and combined. The symptoms must be chronic and have persisted for more than 6 months. Some symptoms should be present before age 7.
   B. A comprehensive, developmentally oriented evaluation should assess the child's functioning within academic and psychosocial contexts.
   C. Findings on sensory, physical, and neurologic examinations are usually normal. Motor coordination, language skills, and social style should be assessed. Behavioral observations should be interpreted cautiously because children may show few symptoms of AD/HD in the office setting.
   D. Laboratory studies, such as a thyroid screen or electroencephalography, should be based on clinical indications. Lead levels and hematocrit should be considered in preschool children.

DSM-IV Diagnostic Criteria for Attention-Deficit Hyperactivity Disorder

At least six of the following symptoms of inattention or hyperactivity-impulsivity must be evident:

Inattention
   Lack of attention to details or careless mistakes in schoolwork or other activities
   Difficulty sustaining attention in tasks or play activities
   Impression of not listening when spoken to directly
   Failure to follow through on instructions or finish schoolwork or duties
   Difficulty organizing tasks and activities
   Avoidance or dislike of tasks that require sustained mental effort (eg, school work or homework)
   Tendency to lose things necessary for tasks or activities (eg, toys, school assignments, pencils, books)
   Distractions by extraneous stimuli
   Forgetfulness in daily activities

Hyperactivity
   Fidgeting with hands or feet or squirming in seat
   Not remaining seated when expected
   Running about or climbing excessively
   Difficulty engaging in leisure activities quietly
   Often "on the go" or "driven by a motor"
   Excessive talking

And/Or

Impulsivity
    Tendency to blurt out answers before questions have been completed
    Difficulty awaiting turn
    Tendency to interrupt or intrude on others (eg, butting into conversations or
        games)

Exclusionary Criteria
A. Some hyperactive-impulsive or inattentive symptoms that caused impairment must have
   been present before age 7.
B. Some impairment from the symptoms must be present in two or more settings (eg, at
   school and at home).
C. There must be clear evidence of clinically significant impairment in social, academic or
   occupational functioning.
D. The symptoms do not occur exclusively during the course of a pervasive developmental
   disorder, schizophrenia, or other psychotic disorder, and are not better accounted for by
   another mental disorder.

II. Treatment of attention deficit/hyperactivity disorder

   A. **Short-acting stimulants.** Methylphenidate (Ritalin) and dextroamphetamine
      (Dexedrine) are two commonly used short-acting stimulants. Onset of action is
      generally rapid, and duration of action is about four hours.
   B. **Long-acting stimulants.** Methylphenidate and dextroamphetamine exist in long-acting
      formulations. These forms have a slower onset of action than the short-acting
      stimulants. Co-administration of a rapid-onset stimulant has a rapid onset of effect,
      and the longer-acting drug can prevent rebound symptoms.
   C. **Amphetamine and dextroamphetamine combination (Adderall)** has a duration
      of action that increases as the initial dose is increased. Adderall can adequately
      treat most patients with ADHD when administered once daily.
   D. **Timed-release methylphenidate (Concerta)** consists of a layer of fast-acting
      methylphenidate around a two-chambered capsule; one chamber contains methylphenidate,
      and the other chamber contains a slowly expanding substance that pushes out
      the methylphenidate. Concerta is designed to provide a 12-hour duration of action
      and is a reliable once-daily medication. It is available in 18-mg, 36-mg and 54-mg
      doses, with 54 mg being the recommended maximal daily dose.

Psychostimulants Used in the Treatment of ADHD

Medication	Available forms	Dose (mg)	Doses per day	Effect duration (hours)
Rapid onset, short duration				
Methylpheni-date (Ritalin)	Tablet: 5, 10, 20 mg (10, 20 mg scored)	Initial: 5 Increment: 5 to 10	2 to 6	1 to 4 hours
Dextroamphet-amine (Dexe-drine)	Capsule: 5, 10, 15 mg	Initial: 2.5 to 5 Increment: 2.5 to 5	1 to 3	1 to 8 hours
(Dextrostat)	Tablet: 5 mg (scored)	Same as above	1 to 3	1 to 8 hours
Dexmethylphe-nidate (Focalin)	2.5, 5, 10 mg	10 mg bid, 4 hours apart	2	6 hours

Medication	Available forms	Dose (mg)	Doses per day	Effect duration (hours)
Slower onset, longer duration				
Methylphenidate (Ritalin-SR)	Tablet: 20 mg	Initial: 20 Increment: 20	1 to 3	3 to 9 hours
(Metadate-ER)	Tablet: 10, 20 mg	Same as above	1 to 3	3 to 9 hours
Dextroamphetamine (Dexedrine Spansules)	Capsule: 5, 10, 15 mg	Initial: 5 Increment: 5	1 to 3	6 to 8 hours
Pemoline (Cylert)	Tablet: 18.75, 37.5 and 75 mg, and 37.5-mg chewable tablet (all scored)	Initial: 37.5 Increment: 18.7	1 to 2	7 to 9 hours
Rapid onset, longer duration				
Amphetamine-dextroamphetamine (Adderall)	Tablet: 5, 7.5, 10, 12.5, 15, 20, 30 mg (scored for halves and quarters)	Initial: 2.5 to 10 Increment: 2.5 to 5	1 to 3	6 to 8 hours
Methylphenidate (Concerta)	Capsule: 18, 36, 54 mg	Initial: 18 Increment: 18	1	12 hours
Methylphenidate (Metadate CD)	Capsule: 18, 36, 54 mg	Initial: 18 Increment: 18	1	12 hours

- **E. Antidepressants.** The tricyclic antidepressants are common additions to treatment when trying to improve the patient's sleep and appetite, or treat a comorbidity of enuresis. If depression is a comorbidity, therapy with a selective serotonin reuptake inhibitors (SSRIs) should be considered. The SSRIs can also be useful in patients who seem to be hyperfocused on certain activities, such as computer games, or who exhibit obsessive-compulsive behaviors.
- **F. Other adjunctive medications.** The alpha$_2$ blockers clonidine (Catapres) and guanfacine (Tenex) are useful in modulating motor tics, anger, irritability, anxiety and frustration. Beta-blockers and low doses of carbamazepine (Tegretol) and divalproex (Depakote) can also be helpful. When extreme oppositional defiant behavior is a suspected comorbidity or when tics remain problematic, therapy with risperidone (Risperdal) could be initiated.
- **G. Behavior modification training.** Effective discipline should target problem behaviors with consistency while minimizing interactions that could damage the child's self-esteem. Behavior modification techniques should emphasize positive reinforcement.

References, see page 164.

Failure to Thrive

Failure to thrive (FTT) is usually first considered when a child is found to weigh less than the third percentile for age and gender. Although FTT occurs in all socioeconomic strata, it is more frequent in families living in poverty. FTT describes a sign; it is not a diagnosis. The underlying etiology must be determined. Ten percent of children seen in the primary care setting show signs of growth failure. Children with FTT attain lower verbal intelligence, poorer language development, less developed reading skills, lower social maturity, and have a higher incidence of behavioral disturbances.

I. Pathophysiology
   A. **Diagnostic criteria for failure to thrive**
      1. A child younger than 2 years of age whose weight is below the 3rd or 5th percentile for age on more than one occasion.
      2. A child younger than 2 years of age whose weight is less than 80% of the ideal weight for age.
      3. A child younger than 2 years of age whose weight crosses two major percentiles downward on a standardized growth grid.
   B. **Exceptions** to the previously noted criteria include the following:
      1. Children of genetically short stature.
      2. Small-for-gestational age infants.
      3. Preterm infants.
      4. "Overweight" infants whose rate of height gain increases while the rate of weight gain decreases.
      5. Infants who are normally lean.
   C. Many patients with FTT have either an organic or nonorganic cause; however, a sizable number of patients have both psychosocial and organic causes for their condition. FTT is a syndrome of malnutrition brought on by a combination of organic, behavioral, and environmental factors.

II. Clinical evaluation of poor weight gain or weight loss
   A. **Feeding history** should assess details of breast or formula feeding, timing and introduction of solids, who feeds the infant, position and placement of the infant for feeding, and stooling or vomiting patterns.
   B. **Developmental history** should cover gestational and perinatal history, developmental milestones, infant temperament, and the infant's daily routine.
   C. **Psychosocial history** should include family composition, employment status, financial status, stress, isolation, child-rearing beliefs, maternal depression, and the caretaker's own history of possible childhood abuse or neglect.
   D. **Family history** should include heights, weights, illnesses, and constitutional short stature, inherited diseases, or developmental delay.

Causes of Inadequate Caloric Intake

Lack of Appetite
- Anemia (eg, iron deficiency)
- Psychosocial problems (eg, apathy)
- Central nervous system (CNS) pathology (eg, hydrocephalus, tumor)
- Chronic infection (eg, urinary tract infection, acquired immunodeficiency syndrome)
- Gastrointestinal disorder (eg, pain from reflux esophagitis)

Difficulty with Ingestion
- Psychosocial problems (eg, apathy, rumination)
- Cerebral palsy/CNS disorder (eg, hypertonia, hypotonia)
- Craniofacial anomalies (eg, choanal atresia, cleft lip and palate micrognathia, glossoptosis)
- Dyspnea (congenital heart disease, pulmonary disease)
- Feeding disorder
- Generalized muscle weakness/pathology (eg, myopathies)
- Tracheoesophageal fistula
- Genetic syndrome (eg, Smith-Lemli-Opitz-syndrome)
- Congenital syndrome (eg, fetal alcohol syndrome)

Unavailability of Food
- Inappropriate feeding technique
- Inadequate volume of food
- Inappropriate food for age
- Withholding of food (abuse, neglect, psychosocial)

Vomiting
- CNS pathology (increased intracranial pressure)
- Intestinal tract obstruction (eg, pyloric stenosis, malrotation)
- Gastroesophageal reflux
- Drugs (eg, syrup of ipecac)

III. **Physical examination**
   A. **Height, weight, and head circumference** should be plotted on a growth curve. Three measurements that are below the 3rd percentile indicate an underlying organic disease. If all three measurements are consistently below the third percentile but show the same rate of increase over a period of time, the infant probably had intrauterine growth retardation. If the child's median age for weight is less than the median age for height, the child may be undernourished.
   B. **Dysmorphic features and physical signs** of central nervous system, pulmonary, cardiac, or gastrointestinal disorders, or signs of neglect or abuse (poor hygiene, unexplained bruises or scars, or inappropriate behavior) should be sought.
   C. **Observation of the infant and caretaker.** While feeding and playing, the infant may avoid eye contact or withdraw from physical attention and may show a poor suck or swallow, or aversion to oral stimulation. Ineffective feeding technique or inappropriate response to the infant's physiologic or social cues may be displayed by the caretaker.
   D. **Diagnostic testing**
      1. **Laboratory testing.** Tests that will usually exclude an organic pathology include a complete blood count, urinalysis, urine culture, blood urea nitrogen, creatinine, serum electrolyte levels, and a tuberculin test.
      2. **Radiologic determination of bone age.** If the bone age is normal, it is unlikely that the infant has a systemic chronic disease or a hormonal abnormality as the cause of poor weight gain.
      3. **Severe malnutrition requires** measurement of albumin, alkaline phosphatase, calcium, and phosphorous to assess protein status and to look for biochemical rickets.
      4. Human immunodeficiency virus screening or a sweat test may be considered.
   E. **A feeding evaluation** by a nutritionist or an occupational therapist may detect a subtle feeding disorder.

Causes of Inadequate Calorie Absorption

Malabsorption
- Biliary atresia or cirrhosis
- Celiac disease
- Cystic fibrosis
- Enzymatic deficiencies
- Food (protein) sensitivity or intolerance
- Immunologic deficiency
- Inflammatory bowel disease

Diarrhea
- Bacterial gastroenteritis
- Parasitic infection

Hepatitis

Hirschsprung Disease

Refeeding diarrhea

Causes of Increased Calorie Requirements

Increased Metabolism/Increased Use of Calories
- Chronic/recurrent infection (eg, urinary tract infection, tuberculosis)
- Chronic respiratory insufficiency (eg, chronic lung disease)
- Congenital heart disease/acquired heart disease
- Malignancy
- Chronic anemia
- Toxins (lead)
- Drugs (eg, excess levothyroxine)
- Endocrine disorders (eg, hyperthyroidism, hyperaldosteronism)

Defective Use of Calories
- Metabolic disorders (eg, aminoacidopathies, inborn errors of carbohydrate metabolism)
- Renal tubular acidosis
- Chronic hypoxemia (eg, cyanotic heart disease)

IV. **Treatment of failure to thrive**
   A. The normal, healthy infant requires an average of 100 kcal/kg of body weight per day. Nutritional requirements in children with FTT usually are 150 kcal/kg per day.
   B. **Treatment of infants**
      1. The number of calories per ounce of formula can be increased by adding less water (13 oz infant formula concentrate mixed with 10 oz water provides 24 kcal/oz high-calorie formula) or by adding more carbohydrate in the form of glucose polymers corn starch or fat in the form of medium-chain triglycerides or corn oil.
      2. Once nutritional recovery begins, the infant often demands and eats enough food to gain weight. At this point, ad libitum oral feedings are appropriate.
   C. **Treatment of older children.** Foods can be fortified with such items as milk products, margarine, oil, and peanut butter.
References, see page 164.

Speech and Language Development

Language is defined as a symbolic system for the storage and exchange of information. Language consists of auditory expressive ability (speech), receptive ability (listening comprehension), and visual communication (gestures).

I. Normal speech and language development
   A. Auditory expressive language development
      1. **In the first 4 to 6 weeks**, the earliest sounds consist of cooing.
      2. **In the first few months**, bilabial sounds begin, consisting of blowing bubbles or the "raspberry."
      3. **By 5 months**, laughing and monosyllables appear, such as "da," "ba," or "ga."
      4. **Between 6 and 8 months**, infants begin polysyllabic babbling, consisting of the same syllable repeated, such as "mamama," "dadadada."
      5. **By 9 months**, infants sporadically say "mama" or "dada" without knowing the meaning of these sounds.
      6. **By 10 months of age**, infants use "mama" and "dada" consistently to label the appropriate parent.
      7. **By 12 months**, infants acquire one or two words other than "mama," or "dada."
      8. **During the second year of life**, vocabulary growth velocity accelerates, starting at one new word per week at 12 months of age and increasing to one or more new words per day by 24 months of age.
      9. **By 18 to 20 months**, a toddler should be using a minimum of 20 words; the 24-month-old should have a vocabulary of at least 50 words.
      10. Early during the **second year of life** toddlers produce jargon, consisting of strings of different sounds, with rising and falling, speech-like inflection. These speech inflection patterns of are referred to as prosody.
      11. **By 24 months of age**, toddlers are producing two-word phrases, such as "want milk!"
      12. **In the second year of life**, pronouns appear ("me" and "you").
      13. **Third year.** Vocabulary growth velocity reaches a rate of several new words per day. A 30-month-old's vocabulary should be too large for the parent to count (>150 words).
      14. **By 24 to 30 months**, children develop "telegraphic" speech, which consists of three- to five-word sentences.
      15. **By 2 years**, the child's speech should be one-half intelligible; by 3 years, it should be three-fourths intelligible, and it should be completely intelligible by age 4 years.
   B. Auditory receptive language development
      1. **Newborn infants** respond to vocal stimuli by eye widening or changes in sucking rate.
      2. **The 2- or 3-month-old infant** watches and listens intently to adults and may vocalize back.
      3. **By 4 months of age** the normal infant will turn his head to locate the source of a voice; turning to inanimate stimuli, such as a bell, occurs 1 month later.
      4. **By 7 to 9 months of age**, an infant will attend selectively to his own name.
      5. **By 9 months of age**, infants comprehend the word "no."
      6. **By 1 year of age**, infants respond to one-step commands such as "Give it to me."
      7. **By 2 years of age**, toddlers can follow novel two-step commands. (eg, "Put away your shoes, then go sit down").
      8. **By 2 years**, children will point to objects on command and name simple objects on command.

     9. By 36 months, a child's receptive vocabulary includes 800 words, expanding to 1500-2000 words by age 5.

     10. By 5 years, children are able to follow three- and four-step commands.

C. Visual language development

  1. During the first few weeks, the infant will display alert visual fixation.

  2. By 4 to 6 weeks, a social smile appears.

  3. By age 4 to 5 months, the infant will turn towards a voice.

  4. By 6 to 7 months, infants play gesture games, such as patty cake and peek-a-boo.

  5. Between 8 and 9 months, infants reciprocate and eventually initiate gesture games.

  6. By 9 months, infants appropriately wave bye-bye on command.

  7. Between 9 and 12 months, infants express their desire for an object by reaching and crying.

  8. By 12 months, infants indicate desired objects by pointing with the index finger.

II. Classification of speech and language disorders

A. Hearing loss

  1. One infant per thousand is born with bilateral, severe-to-profound hearing loss. Two children per thousand are deafened during the first 3 years of life.

  2. One-third of congenital deafness is genetic in origin, one-third is nongenetic, and one-third is of unknown etiology. The most common nongenetic cause of deafness is fetal CMV infection.

B. Mental retardation

  1. Three percent of children are mentally retarded, and all children who are mentally retarded are language-delayed. Mental retardation (MR) is defined as significantly subaverage general intellectual function plus delayed adaptive skills in the first 5 years of life.

  2. Intelligence that is "significantly subaverage" is defined as more than 2 standard deviations (SD) below the mean. "Mild" MR is defined as -2 to -3 SD. Intelligence tests are standardized to a mean score of 100, and mild MR is equivalent to an intelligence quotient (IQ) of 69 to 55. Moderate MR = -3 to -4 SD (IQ 54 to 40), severe MR = -4 to -5 SD (IQ 39 to 25), and below -5 SD is profound MR (IQ <25).

C. Developmental language disorders (DLD)

  1. DLD are disorders characterized by selective impairment of speech and/or language development. General intelligence is normal. DLD affects 5-10% of preschool children, and affected boys outnumber affected girls by 3:1.

  2. In the majority of cases, the etiology of DLD remains unknown; however, DLD can be caused by sex chromosome aneuploidy, fragile X syndrome, neonatal intracranial hemorrhage, fetal alcohol effects, head trauma, or human immunodeficiency virus encephalopathy.

  3. Autism manifests as delayed and deviant language development, impaired affective development, monotonously repetitious behaviors with an insistence on routines, and an onset before 30 months of age. The prevalence is 0.2%. Autism can be caused by most of the same etiologies that cause MR.

  4. Stuttering

    a. Physiologic dysfluency is characterized by a transient loss of normal rate and rhythm of speech, and it is normal in children between 2 and 4 years of age. Physiologic disfluency involves repetition of whole words ("I want . . . I want . . . I want to go home").

    b. Stuttering involves repetition of shorter speech segments ("I wu . . . wu . . . wwwant to go home") or a complete inability to initiate a word, referred to as "blockage." The prevalence peaks at 4% between 2 and 4 years of age and declines to 1% among older children and adults.

      5. Dysarthria is caused by a physical impairment of the muscles of speech production. Dysarthria in children usually is caused by cerebral palsy.

III. **Clinical evaluation of speech and language disorders**

    A. **Infants with hearing-impairment.** Deaf infants coo and babble normally until 6 months of age. Thereafter, vocal output gradually diminishes.

    B. **Mentally retarded children** manifest delay in all language areas. Cooing and babbling may be reduced and delayed.

    C. **Developmental language delay** presents with expressive and receptive impairment, such as impaired intelligibility and delayed emergence of sentence structure. Speech may be effortful and reduced in amount.

    D. **Autistic children** manifest delayed and deviant language, impaired affective development, and repetitious behaviors with an insistence on routines. Autistic type language disorder is marked by impaired pragmatics—failure to use language as a medium of social interaction.

IV. **Diagnostic evaluation of speech and language disorders**

    A. **Developmental testing** by a speech/language pathologist should be undertaken once speech or language delay has been detected.

    B. **Audiologic testing** is indicated for all children with a sign of a speech or language disorder.

    C. **Karyotype and DNA probe studies for fragile X** are indicated in children who have mental retardation, autism, or developmental language disorder.

    D. **Human immunodeficiency virus (HIV) serology** is recommended in higher risk speech-delayed children to exclude HIV encephalopathy.

    E. **Creatine kinase** measurement to exclude Duchenne muscular dystrophy is indicated for boys who have speech delay plus gross motor delay but who do not have increased deep tendon reflexes.

    F. **Cranial MRI** is indicated in the presence of focal neurologic abnormalities or dysmorphic features suggestive of a structural brain abnormality (eg, hypertelorism, midfacial hypoplasia, aberrant hair patterning).

V. **Management of speech and language disorders.** The child who has DLD should be referred for speech therapy. Stuttering requires referral to a speech pathologist. Hearing loss is treated with amplification. Therapy for autism is directed at enhancing communication and social skills.

References, see page 164.

Cardiac Disorders

Heart Murmurs

Ninety percent of children will have an audible heart murmur at some point in time. Normal murmurs include vibratory and pulmonary flow murmurs, venous hums, carotid bruits, and the murmur of physiologic branch pulmonary artery stenosis. Less than 5% of heart murmurs in children are caused by cardiac pathology.

I. **Clinical evaluation of heart murmurs**
    A. Cyanosis, exercise intolerance, feeding difficulties, dyspnea, or syncope signify potential cardiac dysfunction. Failure to thrive, diffuse diaphoresis, unexplained persistent irritability or lethargy, and atypical chest pain also suggest the possibility of organic heart disease.
    B. The majority of children who have heart murmurs are asymptomatic. In early infancy, however, cardiac malformations may manifest as persistent peaceful tachypnea (a respiratory rate greater than 60 breaths/min).
C. **Family history** of a congenital cardiovascular malformation increases the risk of a cardiac defect, such as with DiGeorge syndrome (type B interrupted aortic arch, truncus arteriosus).
    D. **Gestational course** should be reviewed for exposure to teratogens or maternal illnesses. Fetal exposure to lithium may cause Ebstein anomaly of the tricuspid valve. Ventricular and atrial septal defects occur with fetal alcohol syndrome. Transient hypertrophic cardiomyopathy and tetralogy of Fallot are associated with maternal diabetes. Maternal collagen vascular disease may lead to fetal complete heart block.

II. **Physical examination**
    A. **Noncardiac malformations.** Twenty-five percent of children who have heart disease have extracardiac anomalies. Diaphragmatic hernia, tracheoesophageal fistula and esophageal atresia, omphalocele, or imperforate anus are associated with congenital cardiac defects in 15-25% of infants.
    B. **Cyanotic infants or children,** abnormal rate or pattern of breathing, a persistently hyperdynamic precordium, precordial bulging, or asymmetric pulses should be referred to a cardiologist. Signs of congestive heart failure (inappropriate tachycardia, tachypnea, hepatomegaly, abnormal pulse volume) also should prompt referral to a cardiologist.
    C. **Auscultatory criteria signifying cardiac disease**
        1. Loud, pansystolic, late systolic, diastolic, or continuous murmurs; an abnormally loud or single second heart sound
        2. Fourth heart sound or S_4 gallop
        3. Ejection or midsystolic clicks
    D. **Ventricular septal defect (VSD)** is a harsh pansystolic murmur of even amplitude that is audible at the lower left sternal border.
    E. **Patent ductus arteriosus (PDA)** causes a murmur that is continuous, louder in systole, and located at the upper left sternal border.
    F. **Ejection (crescendo-decrescendo) murmurs** are caused by ventricular outflow obstruction. Ejection murmurs begin after the first heart sound.

Characteristics of Organic Murmurs				
Lesion	**Shape**	**Timing**	**Location**	**Other Findings**
Ventricular septal defect	Plateau	Holosystolic	LLSB	Apical mid-diastolic murmur
Mitral regurgitation	Plateau	Holosystolic	Apex	Higher pitched than VSD murmur
Atrial septal defect	Ejection	Systolic	ULSB	Persistent S2 split
Patent ductus arteriosus	Diamond	Continuous	ULSB	Bounding pulses
Aortic valve stenosis	Ejection	Systolic	URSB	Ejection click
Subvalvular aortic stenosis	Ejection	Systolic	ML-URSB	No ejection click
Hypertrophic cardiomyopathy	Ejection	Systolic	LLSB- apex	Laterally displaced PMI
Coarctation	Ejection	Systolic	ULSB-Left back	Pulse disparity
Pulmonary valve stenosis	Ejection	Systolic	ULSB	Ejection click; wide S2 split
Tetralogy of Fallot	Ejection	Systolic	MLSB	Cyanosis

LLSB = lower left sternal border, ULSB = upper left sternal border, URSB = upper right sternal border, MLSB = mid-left sternal border, S2 = second heart sound, PMI = point of maximal impulse.

III. **Differentiation of normal from pathologic murmurs**
   A. **Criteria for diagnosis of a normal heart murmur**
      1. Asymptomatic patient.
      2. No evidence of associated cardiac abnormalities, extracardiac congenital malformations, or syndromes.
      3. Auscultatory features are characteristic of an innocent murmur.

Normal Murmurs					
Type	**Shape**	**Timing**	**Pitch**	**Location**	**Other Findings**
Vibratory	Ejection	Midsystolic	Low	LLSB-apex	Intensity ≤ grade II
Venous hum	Diamond	Continuous	Medium	Subclavicular	Disappears in supine position

Type	Shape	Timing	Pitch	Location	Other Findings
Pulmonary flow	Flow	Systolic	Medium	ULSB	Normal S2 split
Physiologic branch pulmonary artery stenosis	Ejection	Systolic	Medium	Entire chest	Disappears by 4 to 6 months of age

LLSB = lower left sternal border, ULSB = upper left sternal border, S2 = second heart sound.

IV. Heart murmurs in the newborn infant

A. Sixty percent of healthy term newborn infants have normal heart murmurs. One-third of neonates who have serious heart malformations may not have a detectable heart murmur during the first 2 weeks of life. Thirty percent of newborn infants subsequently determined to have heart disease are discharged from the newborn nursery as ostensibly healthy.

B. **Persistent peaceful tachypnea** should not be dismissed; 90% of infants who have serious cardiac disease have persistent tachypnea after birth.

C. **A persistently hyperdynamic precordium** suggests organic heart disease.

D. **Auscultation of the second heart sound.** In healthy neonates, the second heart sound is split audibly by 12 hours of age. A single second heart sound in a quiet neonate indicates: 1) the absence of one outflow tract valve (aortic or pulmonary atresia); 2) an abnormal position of the great vessels (transposition of the great arteries or tetralogy of Fallot); or 3) pulmonary hypertension (ventricular defect, persistent pulmonary hypertension).

References, see page 164.

Chest Pain in Children

Chest pain is the presenting complaint in 6 per 1,000 children who present to pediatric clinics. Young children are more likely to have a cardiorespiratory cause of their pain, such as cough, asthma, pneumonia, or heart disease; adolescents are more likely to have pain associated with a psychogenic disturbance.

I. Differential diagnosis of chest pain in children

A. Cardiac disease

1. Cardiac disease is a rare cause of chest pain in children. However, myocardial infarction can rarely result from anomalous coronary arteries. Some children will have a pansystolic, continuous or mitral regurgitation murmur or gallop rhythm that suggests myocardial dysfunction.

2. Arrhythmias may cause palpitations or abnormalities on cardiac examination. Supraventricular tachycardia is the most common arrhythmia, but premature ventricular beats or tachycardia also can cause episodes of brief sharp chest pain.

3. **Hypertrophic obstructive cardiomyopathy** is an autosomal dominant structural disorder; therefore, there often is a family history of the condition. Children may have a murmur that may be audible when standing or when performing a Valsalva maneuver.

4. **Mitral valve prolapse** may cause chest pain secondary to papillary muscle or endocardial ischemia. A midsystolic click and a late systolic murmur may be detected.
5. **Cardiac infections** are uncommon causes of pediatric chest pain.
    a. **Pericarditis** presents with sharp, stabbing pain that improves when the patient sits up and leans forward. The child usually is febrile; is in respiratory distress; and has a friction rub, distant heart sounds, neck vein distention, and pulsus paradoxus.
    b. **Myocarditis** presents as mild pain that has been present for several days. After a few days of fever, vomiting and lightheadedness, the patient may develop pain or shortness of breath on exertion. Examination may reveal muffled heart sounds, fever, a gallop rhythm, or tachycardia.
    c. **Chest radiography** will show cardiomegaly in both of these infections, and the electrocardiogram will be abnormal. An echocardiogram will confirm the diagnosis.

B. **Musculoskeletal pain**
    1. Musculoskeletal pain is one of the most common diagnoses in children who have chest discomfort. Children frequently strain chest wall muscles while exercising.
    2. **Trauma** to the chest may result in a mild contusion or a rib fracture. The physical examination will reveal chest tenderness.
    3. **Costochondritis** is common in children, and it is characterized by tenderness over the costochondral junctions. The pain is sharp and exaggerated by physical activity or breathing.

C. **Respiratory conditions**
    1. **Severe cough, asthma, or pneumonia** may cause chest pain because of overuse of chest wall muscles. Crackles, wheezes, tachypnea, or decreased breath sounds are present.
    2. **Exercise-induced asthma** may cause chest pain, which can be confirmed with a treadmill test.
    3. **Spontaneous pneumothorax or pneumomediastinum** may occasionally cause chest pain with respiratory distress. Children with asthma, cystic fibrosis or Marfan syndrome are at high risk. Signs include respiratory distress, decreased breath sounds on the affected side, and palpable subcutaneous air.
    4. **Pulmonary embolism** is extremely rare in pediatric patients, but it should be considered in the adolescent girl who has dyspnea, fever, pleuritic pain, cough, and hemoptysis. Oral contraceptives or recent abortion increase the risk. Young males who have had recent leg trauma also are at risk.

D. **Psychogenic chest pain** may present with hyperventilation or an anxious appearance. A recent stressful event (separation from friends, parental divorce, school failure) may often be related temporally to the onset of the chest pain.

E. **Gastrointestinal disorders**
    1. **Reflux esophagitis** often causes chest pain, which is described as burning, substernal, and worsened by reclining or eating spicy foods. This condition is confirmed with a therapeutic trial of antacids.
    2. **Foreign body ingestion** may cause chest pain when the object lodges in the esophagus. A radiograph confirms the diagnosis.

F. **Miscellaneous causes of pediatric chest pain**
    1. **Sickle cell disease** may cause an acute chest syndrome.
    2. **Marfan syndrome** may cause chest pain and fatal abdominal aortic aneurysm dissection.
    3. **Collagen vascular disorders** may cause chest pain and pleural effusions.
    4. **Shingles** may cause chest pain that precedes or occurs simultaneously with

the rash.
5. **Coxsackievirus infection** may lead to pleurodynia with paroxysms of sharp chest pain.
6. **Breast tenderness during puberty or early breast changes of pregnancy** may present as chest pain.
7. **Idiopathic chest pain.** No diagnosis can be determined in 20-45% of cases of pediatric chest pain.

I. Clinical evaluation of chest pain
A. **A history and physical examination** will reveal the etiology of chest pain in most cases. The history may reveal asthma, previous heart disease, or Kawasaki disease. Family history may reveal familial hypertrophic obstructive cardiomyopathy.
B. **The frequency and severity of the pain** and whether the pain interrupts the child's daily activity should be determined. Pain that wakes the child from sleep is more likely to be related to an organic etiology.
C. **Burning pain** in the sternal area suggests esophagitis. Sharp stabbing pain that is relieved by sitting up and leaning forward suggests pericarditis in a febrile child.
D. **Mode of onset of pain.** Acute onset of pain is more likely to represent an organic etiology. Chronic pain is much more likely to have a idiopathic or psychogenic origin.
E. **Precipitating factors**
   1. **Trauma, muscle strain or choking on a foreign body** should be sought.
   2. **Exercise-induced chest pain** may be caused by cardiac disease or exercise-induced asthma.
   3. **Syncope, fever or palpitations** associated with chest pain are signs of an organic etiology.
   4. **Joint pain, rash or fever** may be suggested by the presence of collagen vascular disease.
   5. **Stressful conditions** at home or school should be sought.
   6. **Substance abuse (cocaine) or oral contraceptives** should be sought in adolescents.
F. **Physical examination**
   1. **Severe distress** warrants immediate treatment for life-threatening conditions, such as pneumothorax.
   2. **Hyperventilation** may be distinguished from respiratory distress by the absence of cyanosis or nasal flaring.
   3. **Pallor or poor growth** may suggest a malignancy or collagen vascular disease.
   4. **Abdominal tenderness** may suggest abdominal pain that is referred to the chest.
   5. **Rales, wheezes, decreased breath sounds, murmurs, rubs, muffled heart sounds or arrhythmias** suggest a cardiopulmonary pathology.
   6. **The chest wall** should be evaluated for bruises (trauma), tenderness (musculoskeletal pain), or subcutaneous air (pneumothorax or pneumomediastinum).

II. Laboratory evaluation
A. **A chest radiograph** is warranted if the patient has fever, respiratory distress, or abnormal breath sounds. Fever and cardiomegaly suggests pericarditis or myocarditis.
B. **Electrocardiography** is recommended if the pain was acute in onset (began in the last 2-3 days) or if there is an abnormal cardiac examination (unexplained tachycardia, arrhythmia, murmur, rub, or click).
C. **Exercise stress testing or pulmonary function testing** is appropriate for evaluation of cardiac disease or asthma.
D. **Holter monitoring** is warranted for syncope or palpitations.

    E. Children with chronic pain, a normal physical examination, and no history suggestive of cardiac or pulmonary disease do not require laboratory studies.

    F. Blood counts and sedimentation rates are of value if collagen vascular disease infection, or malignancy is suspected.

    G. Drug screening may be indicated in the older child who has acute pain associated with anxiety, tachycardia, hypertension, or shortness of breath.

IV.   **Management of pediatric chest pain**

    A. Emergency department referral is necessary if the child is in severe distress or has a history of significant trauma.

    B. Referral to a cardiologist is recommended for children with known or suspected heart disease, syncope, palpitations, or pain on exertion.

    C. Musculoskeletal, psychogenic or idiopathic pain usually will respond to reassurance analgesics, rest, and application of a heating pad. If esophagitis is suspected a trial of antacids may be beneficial.

References, see page 164.

Allergic and Dermatologic Disorders

Asthma

Asthma affects about 5 percent of the population younger than 18 years. Fifty to 80 percent of children with asthma develop symptoms before five years of age.

Diagnosis

A. **Symptoms of asthma** include episodic or persistent coughing, wheezing, shortness of breath, rapid breathing or chest tightness. Symptoms tend to be worse during the evening or early morning hours, or are associated with triggers (eg, exercise, allergen exposure). Wheezing may also be caused by respiratory infections, rhinitis, sinusitis or vocal cord dysfunction. Foreign body aspiration, cystic fibrosis or heart disease may also cause wheezing.

B. **Factors associated with asthma** include allergy, family history of asthma or allergy, perinatal exposure to tobacco smoke, viral respiratory infections, male gender and low birth weight. Young children who develop persistent asthma are likely to have increased serum IgE levels, atopic dermatitis and rhinitis, severe lower respiratory infections, and diminished airway function.

C. **Symptom patterns, severity of symptoms** and precipitating factors should be assessed: "How often and when do episodes occur?" "What is their duration?" "Do symptoms occur or worsen during the night, with exercise or with an infection?" "Are they precipitated or aggravated by specific triggers?" "Do they interfere with sleep or daily activities, or require emergency department or hospital visits?" "How often are short-acting bronchodilators used?" "Are symptoms temporarily relieved by bronchodilators?"

D. **Pulmonary function tests** should be conducted to confirm the diagnosis. Spirometry performed before and 15 to 20 minutes after the child inhales a short-acting bronchodilator assesses airflow obstruction. Pulmonary function results consistent with asthma include variable airflow obstruction (20 percent or more), and an increase in forced expiratory volume in one second (FEV_1) of 12 percent or more after bronchodilator therapy. Routine pulmonary function testing is unreliable in infants and many preschool children.

Diagnosis of Asthma

Asthma diagnosis	Days with symptoms*	Nights with symptoms	PEF (% personal best) or FEV_2 (% predicted best)
Step 4: severe persistent	Continual	Frequent	≤ 60
Step 3: moderate persistent	Daily	≥ 5 times per month	>60 to <80
Step 2: mild persistent	>2 times per week	3 to 4 times per month	≥ 80
Step 1: mild intermittent	≥ 2 times per week	≤ 2 per month	≥ 80

II. Treatment

A. Triggers and environmental control

1. Asthma triggers include dust mites or mold spores, animal dander, cockroaches, pollen, indoor and outdoor pollutants, tobacco smoke, smoke from wood-burning, perfumes, cleaning agents, aspirin or other nonsteroidal anti-inflammatory drugs, beta-blockers, exercise, hyperventilation, cold air, stress, gastroesophageal reflux, respiratory infection).

2. Environmental control measures include removing carpets, weekly washing of bedding and clothing in hot water, use of mattress and pillow covers, removing stuffed animals, keeping pets outdoors and using special furnace filters.

3. Up to 80 percent of asthmatic children have allergic rhinitis. If specific IgE hypersensitivity has been identified by radioallergosorbent test (RAST) or skin testing, the triggers to be avoided can be specified. Exposure to tobacco smoke should be strictly avoided.

Stepwise Approach for Managing Asthma

Asthma	Quick relief	Long-term control	Medication
Step 4: severe, persistent	Short-acting bronchodilator as needed: • Inhaled short-acting beta$_2$ agonist or • Oral beta$_2$ agonist	Daily anti-inflammatory medications: • High-dose inhaled corticosteroid and • If needed, add systemic corticosteroids (0.25 to 2 mg per kg per day) and reduce to lowest dosage.	Oral corticosteroids: Methylprednisone (Medrol), 2-mg tablet Prednisolone (Prelone syrup), 5 mg per 5 mL (Pediapred liquid), 5 mg per 5 mL. Prednisone 5-mg tablet (Deltasone), 5-mg tab (Intensol), 5 mg/mL liquid
Step 3: moderate, persistent	Short-acting bronchodilator as needed: • Inhaled short-acting beta$_2$ agonist by nebulizer or spacer and face mask or • Oral beta$_2$ agonist	Daily anti-inflammatory medications, either: • High-dose inhaled corticosteroid or, once control is established • Low- to medium-dose inhaled corticosteroid and long-acting bronchodilator (eg, long-acting inhaled beta$_2$ agonist or theophylline SR)	Short-acting beta$_2$ agonist Albuterol (Airet nebulizer), 2.5 mg in 3 mL q4-6h PRN (Proventil-HFA MDI) 2 puffs q4-6h PRN (Ventolin Rotacaps DPI), 1-2 caps q4-6h PRN Long-acting beta2 agonist Salmeterol (Serevent MDI, Serevent Diskus DPI) 2 puffs q12h; 1 inhalation q12h Albuterol SR (Volmax tablet, Proventil Repetabs) 4-8 mg bid Salmeterol/Fluticasone (Advair Diskus) 100 µg/50 µg 250 µg/50 µg 500 µg/50 µg 1 puff q12h

Stepwise Approach for Managing Asthma

Asthma	Quick relief	Long-term control	Medication
Step 2: mild, persistent	Short-acting bronchodilator as needed: • Inhaled short-acting beta$_2$ agonist or • Oral beta$_2$ agonist	Daily anti-inflammatory medications	**Inhaled corticosteroids** • Beclomethasone (Beclovent MDI) 4-8 puffs bid (Vanceril DS MDI) 2-4 puffs bid • Budesonide (Pulmicort Turbuhaler DPI)1-2 inhalations bid. Pulmicort Respules, 0.25 mg, 0.5 mg. 1-2 bid. • Flunisolide (AeroBid MDI) 2-4 puffs bid • Fluticasone (Flovent), 2-4 puffs bid (Flovent Rotadisk) 1 bid. • Triamcinolone (Azmacort MDI) 4 puffs bid. **Theophylline** 200 mg, 300 mg (SR), 450 mg (TR). 100-300 mg bid **Antileukotrienes** • Zafirlukast (Accolate), 10-mg tablet, 20 mg bid • Montelukast (Singulair), 4- or 5-mg chewable tab, 10 mg qhs • Zileuton (Zyflo Flimtab), 600-mg tab, 600 mg qid • Cromolyn (Intal) inhaler, 2-4 puffs tid-qid • Nedocromil (Tilade) inhaler, 2-4 puffs bid-qid
Step 1: mild, intermittent	Short-acting bronchodilator as needed <2 times per week: • Inhaled, short-acting beta$_2$ agonist or • Oral beta$_2$ agonist	No daily medication	**Short-acting beta$_2$ agonist** Albuterol (Airet nebulizer), 2.5 mg in 3 mL q4-6h PRN (Proventil-HFA MDI) 2 puffs q4-6h PRN (Ventolin Rotacaps DPI), 1-2 caps q4-6h PRN

Drugs for Asthma

Drug	Formulation	Dosage
Inhaled beta$_2$-adrenergic agonists, short-acting		
Albuterol *Proventil* *Proventil-HFA* *Ventolin* *Ventolin Rotacaps*	metered-dose inhaler (90 µg/puff) dry-powder inhaler (200 µg/inhalation)	2 puffs q4-6h PRN 1-2 capsules q4-6h PRN
Albuterol *Proventil* multi-dose vials *Ventolin Nebules* *Ventolin*	nebulized	2.5 mg q4-6h PRN
Levalbuterol - *Xopenex*	nebulized	0.63-1.25 mg q6-8h PRN
Inhaled beta2-adrenergic agonist, long-acting		
Formoterol - *Foradil*	dry-powder inhaler (12 µg/puff)	1 puff bid.
Salmeterol *Serevent* *Serevent Diskus*	metered-dose inhaler (21 µg/puff) dry-powder inhaler (50 µg/inhalation)	2 puffs q12h 1 inhalation q12h
Fluticasone/Salmeterol *Advair Diskus*	dry-powder inhaler (100, 250 or 500 µg/puff)	1 puff q12h
Inhaled Corticosteroids		
Beclomethasone dipropionate *Beclovent* *Vanceril* Vanceril Double-Strength	metered-dose inhaler (42 µg/puff) (84 µg/puff)	4-8 puffs bid 2-4 puffs bid
Budesonide *Pulmicort Turbuhaler*	dry-powder inhaler (200 µg/inhalation)	1-2 inhalations bid
Flunisolide - *AeroBid*	metered-dose inhaler (250 µg/puff)	2-4 puffs bid
Fluticasone Flovent *Flovent Rotadisk*	metered-dose inhaler (44, 110 or 220 µg/puff) dry-powder inhaler (50, 100 or 250 µg/inhalation)	2-4 puffs bid (44 µg/puff) 1 inhalation bid (100 µg/inhalation)
Triamcinolone acetonide *Azmacort*	metered-dose inhaler (100 µg/puff)	2 puffs tid-qid or 4 puffs bid
Leukotriene Modifiers		
Montelukast - *Singulair*	tablets	10 mg qhs

Drug	Formulation	Dosage
Zafirlukast - *Accolate*	tablets	20 mg bid
Zileuton - *Zyflo*	tablets	600 mg qid
Mast Cell Stabilizers		
Cromolyn *Intal*	metered-dose inhaler (800 µg/puff)	2-4 puffs tid-qid
Nedocromil *Tilade*	metered-dose inhaler (1.75 mg/puff)	2-4 puffs bid-qid
Phosphodiesterase Inhibitor		
Theophylline *Slo-Bid Gyrocaps, Theo-Dur, Unidur*	extended-release capsules or tablets	100-300 mg bid

B. Pharmacologic therapy

1. Asthma is classified into four levels of severity: mild intermittent, mild persistent, moderate persistent or severe persistent.
2. The National Asthma Education and Prevention Program guidelines recommend a stepwise approach to pharmacologic treatment starting with the most aggressive therapy necessary to achieve control, followed by a "step down" to the minimal therapy that will maintain control.
3. **Quick-relief medications**
   a. These drugs, including short-acting inhaled or oral beta$_2$ agonists, short-course oral corticosteroids, are taken as needed for immediate relief of acute symptoms.
   b. Short-acting beta$_2$ agonists rapidly relax bronchial smooth muscle and are the therapy of choice to relieve acute symptoms. Beta$_2$ agonists do not affect the underlying disease.
   c. Oral corticosteroids have broad anti-inflammatory effects and may be used in a limited, short course (three to 10 days) to gain initial control.
4. **Long-term control medications.** Medications for long-term control should be taken daily to maintain control.
   a. **Inhaled corticosteroids** are the most effective long-term anti-inflammatory medications. Some corticosteroids are effective in once- or twice-daily dosing regimens. Budesonide inhalation suspension (Pulmicort Respules) is the only nebulizable corticosteroid for children one to eight years. It is available in unit doses of 0.25 mg and 0.50 mg for once- or twice-daily dosing.
   b. **Long-acting beta$_2$ agonists** are not as effective as inhaled corticosteroids. However, long-acting beta$_2$ agonists may be used as add-on therapy with inhaled corticosteroids to reduce nocturnal asthma symptoms and prevent exercise-induced bronchospasm. They should not be used to treat patients with acute symptoms or exacerbations. A long-acting beta$_2$ agonist, salmeterol (Serevent), may provide 24-hour bronchodilation with twice-daily dosing and may reduce nocturnal asthma symptoms. A combination of Salmeterol and fluticasone (Advair Diskus) is taken as one inhalation twice daily.
   c. **Theophylline** produces mild-to-moderate bronchodilation and may be used as add-on therapy with anti-inflammatory medications. However, theophylline has a narrow therapeutic index, drug interactions and serious side effects. Theophylline is reserved for the treatment of severe asthma, when polypharmacy

is necessary.
   d. **Cromolyn sodium (Intal) and nedocromil (Tilade)** are first-line, daily anti-inflammatory inhaled agents that inhibit bronchoconstriction, with virtually no serious side effects. Frequent administration is required (up to four doses daily), and these agents are less effective than corticosteroids. Nedocromil's bitter taste discourages compliance.
   e. **Antileukotriene agents.** The leukotriene receptor antagonists **montelukast (Singulair)** and **zafirlukast (Accolate)**, and the 5-lipoxygenase inhibitor **zileuton (Zyflo)** target inflammation. Montelukast is available at a dosage of 5 mg once daily at bedtime. A 10-mg tablet is approved for use in children older than 15 years, and a 4- or 5-mg chewable tablet for children two to five years. Zafirlukast is also FDA-labeled for the treatment of children older than seven years, at a dosage of 10 mg twice daily. Zileuton is prescribed infrequently because of hepatotoxicity.

References, see page 164.

Atopic Dermatitis and Eczema

Atopic dermatitis is a chronic inflammation of the skin that occurs in persons of all ages but is more common in children. Atopic dermatitis affects 10 percent of children. The symptoms of atopic dermatitis resolve by adolescence in 50 percent of affected children.

I. **Diagnosis**
   A. Exposure to aeroallergens, irritating chemicals, foods and emotional stress may worsen the rash.
   B. Acute lesions are papules and vesicles on a background of erythema. Subacute lesions may develop scales and lichenification. Chronically involved areas become thick and fibrotic. Lesions can develop secondary infections with crusting and weeping. Xerosis (dry skin) is characteristic.

Diagnostic Features of Atopic Dermatitis

Major features
Pruritus
Chronic or relapsing dermatitis
Personal or family history of atopic disease
Typical distribution and morphology of atopic dermatitis rash:
   Facial and extensor surfaces in infants and young children
   Flexure lichenification in older children and adults

Minor features

Eyes	
Cataracts (anterior subcapsular)	Nipple eczema
Keratoconus	Positive type I hypersensitivity skin tests
Infraorbital folds affected	Propensity for cutaneous infections
Facial pallor	Elevated serum IgE level
Palmar hyperlinearity	Food intolerance
Xerosis	Impaired cell-mediated immunity
Pityriasis alba	Erythroderma
White dermatographism	Early age of onset
Ichthyosis	
Keratosis pilaris	
Nonspecific dermatitis of the hands and feet	

C. In infants and young children, pruritus commonly is present on the scalp, face (cheeks and chin) and extensor surfaces of the extremities. Older children and adults typically have involvement of the flexor surfaces (antecubital and popliteal fossa), neck, wrists and ankles.

D. Exposure to pollens, molds, mites and animal dander may be important in some patients.

II. Treatment

A. **Bathing and moisturizers.** Bathing should occur once daily with warm water for five to 10 minutes. Soap should not be used unless it is needed for the removal of dirt. A mild cleanser (eg, Dove, Basis, Kiss My Face or Cetaphil) may be used. After bathing, patients should apply a moisturizer liberally (eg, Vaseline, Aquaphor, Eucerin, Moisturel, mineral oil or baby oil). Ointments are superior to creams. Lotions are least effective because of their alcohol content.

B. To avoid injury to the skin from scratching, fingernails should be cut short, and cotton gloves can be worn at night.

C. Pruritus that is refractory to moisturizers and conservative measures can be treated with sedating agents such as hydroxyzine (Atarax) and diphenhydramine (Benadryl). Tricyclic antidepressants such as doxepin (Sinequan) and amitriptyline (Elavil) also induce sleep and reduce pruritus.

D. Systemic corticosteroids should be reserved for use in patients with severe treatment-resistant atopic dermatitis.

E. It is reasonable to use a mild topical steroid initially in infants and for intertriginous areas in patients of any age. If the dermatitis is severe, a more potent steroid is needed.

Commonly Used Topical Corticosteroids	
Preparation	Size
Low-Potency Agents	
Hydrocortisone ointment, cream, 1, 2.5% (Hytone)	30 g
Mild-Potency Agents	
Alclometasone dipropionate cream, ointment, 0.05% (Aclovate)	60 g
Triamcinolone acetonide cream, 0.1% (Aristocort)	60 g
Fluocinolone acetonide cream, 0.01% (Synalar)	60 g
Medium-Potency Agents	
Triamcinolone acetonide ointment (Aristocort A), 0.1%	60 g
Betamethasone dipropionate cream (Diprosone), 0.05%	45 g
Mometasone cream 0.1% (Elocon)	45 g
Fluocinolone acetonide ointment, 0.025% (Synalar)	60 g
Betamethasone valerate cream, 0.1% (Valisone)	45 g
Hydrocortisone valerate cream, ointment, 0.2% (Westcort)	60 g

F. Immunosuppressants and antineoplastics
1. **Pimecrolimus (Elidel)** is a non-steroid cream for the treatment of mild to moderate eczema. Pimecrolimus has anti-inflammatory activity. It does not cause skin atrophy. Topical application is comparable to that of a potent topical steroid. 1% pimecrolimus cream is applied twice daily. It may be used in children ≥2 years old.
2. **Tacrolimus (Protopic)** is more potent than pimecrolimus in the treatment of severe or refractory atopic dermatitis, with few adverse effects. Tacrolimus is available in 0.1% and 0.03%. The lower strength may be used in children ≥2 years old.
3. **Cyclosporine (Sandimmune)** has been effective in patients with refractory atopic dermatitis. The condition returns after the cessation of therapy, although not always at the original level of severity.

References, see page 164.

Contact Dermatitis

Contact dermatitis is an extremely common in the pediatric age group. There are two major forms of contact dermatitis: irritant and allergic. Common causes of irritant contact dermatitis include overbathing, drooling, prolonged contact with moisture and feces in the diaper, and bubble baths.

I. **Clinical evaluation**
   A. Contact dermatitis usually first appears in infants 2-6 months of age. Infants and children have rashes on the shoulders, chest, abdomen, and back. Infants usually also have a rash on the face, scalp and around the ears. Children older than 18 months old tend to have rashes on the neck and antecubital and popliteal fossae. Contact dermatitis usually resolves by puberty, but it sometimes recurs at times of stress.
   B. Acute lesions are itchy, red, edematous papules and small vesicles which may progress to weeping and crusting lesions. Chronic rubbing and scratching may cause lichenification and hyperpigmentation.
   C. Patch testing is useful for evaluation of persistent, localized reactions. It also may be useful in patients who have atopic dermatitis and experience a flare or persistence of disease despite appropriate therapy.

II. **Treatment of contact dermatitis**
   A. **Moisture.** Avoidance of excessive bathing, hand washing, and lip licking is recommended. Showers or baths should be limited to no more than 5 minutes. After bathing, patients should apply a moisturizer (Aquaphor, Eucerin, Vaseline) to noninflamed skin.
   B. **Contact with irritants**
      1. Overuse of soap should be discouraged. Use of nonirritating soaps (eg, Dove, Ivory, Neutrogena) should be limited to the axilla, groin, hands, and feet.
      2. Infants often have bright red exudative contact dermatitis (slobber dermatitis) on the cheeks, resulting from drooling. A corticosteroid will usually bring improvement.
   C. **Topical corticosteroids**
      1. Corticosteroid ointments maintain skin hydration and maximize penetration. Corticosteroid creams may sting when applied to acute lesions.
      2. Mid- and low-potency topical corticosteroids are used twice daily for chronic, atopic dermatitis. High-potency steroids may be used for flare-ups, but the potency should be tapered after the dermatitis is controlled.
      3. Use of high-potency agents on the face, genitalia and skinfolds may cause

epidermal atrophy ("stretch marks"), rebound erythema, and susceptibility to bruising.

Commonly Used Topical Corticosteroids	
Preparation	Size
Low-Potency Agents	
Hydrocortisone ointment, cream, 1, 2.5% (Hytone)	30 g
Mild-Potency Agents	
Alclometasone dipropionate cream, ointment, 0.05% (Aclovate)	60 g
Triamcinolone acetonide cream, 0.1% (Aristocort)	60 g
Fluocinolone acetonide cream, 0.01% (Synalar)	60 g
Medium-Potency Agents	
Triamcinolone acetonide ointment (Aristocort A), 0.1%	60 g
Betamethasone dipropionate cream (Diprosone), 0.05%	45 g
Mometasone cream 0.1% (Elocon)	45 g
Fluocinolone acetonide ointment, 0.025% (Synalar)	60 g
Hydrocortisone butyrate 0.1% cream, ointment (Locoid)	45 g
Betamethasone valerate cream, 0.1% (Valisone)	45 g
Hydrocortisone valerate cream, ointment, 0.2% (Westcort)	60 g
High-Potency Agents	
Amcinonide ointment, 0.1% (Cyclocort)	60 g
Betamethasone dipropionate ointment (Diprosone) 0.05%	45 g
Fluocinonide cream, ointment, 0.05% (Lidex)	60 g

4. **Allergic reactions to topical corticosteroids** may occur. Mometasone (Elocon) is the least likely to cause an allergic reaction.
D. **Antihistamines**, such as diphenhydramine or hydroxyzine (Atarax), are somewhat useful for pruritus and are sedating. Nonsedating antihistamines, such as cetirizine (Zyrtec), loratadine (Claritin) and fexofenadine (Allegra), are helpful.
E. **Systemic corticosteroids** are reserved for severe, widespread reactions to poison ivy, or for severe involvement of the hands, face, or genitals. Prednisone, 1-2 mg/kg, is given PO and tapered over 10-18 days.
References, see page 164.

Diaper Dermatitis

Diaper rash occurs in 50% of infants, with 5% having severe rash. The peak incidence is between 9 and 12 months of age.

I. **Pathophysiology**. Breast fed infants have fewer diaper rashes than formula-fed infants. The frequency and severity of diaper dermatitis are significantly lower when the number of diaper changes per day is eight or more. Superabsorbent disposable diapers significantly reduce the severity of diaper rash when compared to cloth diapers.

II. **Classification of diaper dermatitis**
   A. **Dermatoses related to diaper wearing**
      1. **Irritant diaper dermatitis** is the most common form of diaper dermatitis. It is accentuated on the convex areas, including the buttocks, lower abdomen, genitalia, and upper thigh, sparing the creases. It varies in severity from mild erythema (with or without scales) to papules and macerated lesions.
         a. **Management**
            (1) Irritant diaper dermatitis can best be prevented by keeping the skin in the diaper area protected from urine and feces by increasing the frequency of diaper changes and by using superabsorbent disposable diapers.
            (2) A low-potency corticosteroid ointment (hydrocortisone 1%) should be applied four times daily with diaper changes. Anticandidal agents such as nystatin (Mycostatin), clotrimazole (Lotrimin), or ketoconazole (Nizoral) should also be added.
            (3) Thickly applied barrier creams, such as A&D ointment, zinc oxide pastes or Vaseline, may be helpful.
      2. **Candidal diaper dermatitis**
         a. Candidal diaper dermatitis is characterized by beefy red plaques with white scales and satellite papules and pustules, which almost always involve the inguinal creases. It often develops after an episode of diarrhea. KOH scrapings may demonstrate pseudohyphae.
         b. Candidiasis is treated with topical nystatin (Mycostatin), clotrimazole (Lotrimin), miconazole (Monistat), or ketoconazole (Nizoral) applied 3-4 times daily. Hydrocortisone 1% ointment may help decrease erythema and inflammation and can be applied at the same time. Oral nystatin (Mycostatin) suspension, four times a day, should be used if repeated episodes of candidal dermatitis occur. The mother should be evaluated for candidal infection of the nipples or genital tract. In severe cases, oral fluconazole (Diflucan) 3 mg/kg per day as a pulse dose weekly x 2 or for a short course of 5 to 7 days may be of benefit.

References, see page 164.

Dermatophyte Infections

Dermatophytes constitute a group of about 40 fungal species that cause superficial infections called dermatophytoses, ringworm, or tinea.

I. **Tinea capitis**
   A. Tinea capitis presents as inflammation with hair breakage and loss. Inflammatory changes can range from minimal scaling and redness that resembles mild seborrhea to tenderness, redness, edema, purulence, and hair loss (kerion).

    B. A hypersensitivity reaction to fungal antigen can develop, called a dermatophytid or "id" reaction. Id reactions can present with either a dermatitis that includes redness, superficial edema involving the epidermis, and scaling or with a "pityriasis rosea-like" reaction that involves red, scaly papules and ovoid plaques on the face, neck, trunk, and proximal extremities.

    C. Topical antifungals are not effective for hair infection. Griseofulvin is preferred for initial treatment at a starting dose of about 20 mg/kg per day.

    D. Selenium sulfide shampoo (Selsun Blue) is used in conjunction with oral antifungals to reduce contagion. Tinea capitis is contagious until after 2 weeks of systemic treatment. Dermatophytid reactions can be treated with topical corticosteroids.

II. Tinea corporis (ring worm) and tinea cruris

    A. Dermatophyte infection of the body surface is termed tinea corporis. Tinea cruris describes infection of the upper thigh and inguinal area. Examination reveals red, scaly papules and small plaques. These progressively enlarge to form expanding rings, arcs, or annular patterns.

    B. Clearing in previously affected areas produces the typical "ringworm" appearance. Topical therapy is the initial treatment approach.

III.   Tinea pedis and tinea manuum

    A. Tinea pedis infection is often interdigital and is induced by the warmth and moisture of wearing shoes. The web spaces become red and scaly. Fungal infection frequently spreads to involve the soles of the feet or the palms, with dry scale and minimal redness. Scaling extends to the side of the foot or hand. Vesicle and blister formation and itching are common.

    B. Dermatophyte infection often leads to secondary bacterial infection. A dermatophytid reaction may occur, as described for tinea capitis.

    C. Dermatophyte hand infection presents as dry scale on the palm. Infection of just one hand in conjunction with infection of both feet is the most common pattern.

    D. Topical therapy and keeping the involved areas as dry as possible is recommended for hand or foot tinea. Oral therapy may be necessary for recalcitrant disease.

IV.   Onychomycosis (tinea unguium)

    A. Dermatophyte infection of the nail plate is referred to as onychomycosis, characterized by dystrophy of the nail, discoloration, ridging, thickening, fragility, breakage, accumulation of debris beneath the distal aspect of the nail and little or no inflammation.

    B. Oral treatment is required to clear infection, but recurrence is very common.

V. Diagnosis

    A. Potassium hydroxide (KOH) examination of scale, hair, or nail is the most rapid diagnostic method. A sample of scale, hair, or nail from a possibly infected area is placed on a glass slide, covered with a few drops of 30% KOH, and gently heated. The specimen is examined for spores and/or fungal hyphae.

    B. Fungal culture of scale and affected hair or nail can be accomplished by incubation at room temperature for 2 to 3 weeks.

VI.   Treatment

    A. Oral griseofulvin is effective and safe for treatment of tinea capitis in children. However, its erratic oral absorption necessitates doses of about 20 mg/kg per day of the liquid preparation, always administered with a fatty meal or beverage (such as milk). Ultramicrosize griseofulvin can be administered at the lower dose of 8 to 10 mg/kg per day.

    B. Treatment should be continued for 8 to 12 weeks. Liver function testing is not required when griseofulvin is used for 6 months or less. Adverse effects associated with griseofulvin include headaches and gastrointestinal upset.

Systemic Antifungal Agents

Griseofulvin 20 mg/kg per day of microsize liquid or 7 to 10 mg/kg per day of ultramicrosize tablets. Microsize: Cap: 250 mg, susp: 125 mg/5 mL, tab: 250, 500 mg
Ultramicrosize: Tab: 125, 165, 250, 330 mg

Itraconazole (Sporanox) 4 to 6 mg/kg per day. Cap: 100 mg, soln: 10 mg/mL

Terbinafine (Lamisil) 3 to 5 mg/kg per day. Tab: 250 mg

Topical Treatments for Tinea Pedis, Tinea Cruris and Tinea Corporis

Antifungal agent	Prescription	Cream	Solution or spray	Lotion	Powder	Frequency of application
Imidazoles						
Clotrimazole 1 percent (Lotrimin, Mycelex)		X	X	X		Twice daily
Miconazole 2 percent (Micatin, Monistat-Derm)		X	X	X	X	Twice daily
Econazole 1 percent (Spectazole)	X	X				Once daily
Ketoconazole 2 percent (Nizoral)	X	X	X			Once daily
Oxiconazole 1 percent (Oxistat)	X	X		X		Once daily or twice daily
Allylamines						
Naftifine 1 percent (Naftin)	X	X				Once daily or twice daily
Terbinafine 1 percent (Lamisil)	X	X	X			Once daily or twice daily
Butenafine 1 percent (Mentax)		X				Once daily or twice daily

    C. Itraconazole (Sporanox) is effective and can be given orally at 3 to 5 mg/kg per day for 4 to 6 weeks or until clearing, followed by a 4-week period off of therapy. A liquid formulation is available. Cap: 100 mg, soln: 10 mg/mL

    D. Terbinafine (Lamisil) orally at 3 to 6 mg/kg per day for 4 to 6 weeks is effective.

Tab: 250 mg
- **E. Topical antifungals** can be used once to twice daily to clear infections other than tinea capitis and onychomycosis. Newer, more potent topical agents with once-daily dosing can improve compliance.
- **F. Hydrocortisone** 1% or 2.5% can be added to antifungal therapy to reduce inflammation. Affected areas should be kept as cool and as dry as possible.

References, see page 164.

Herpes Simplex Virus Infections

HSV is a member of the herpesvirus family, which includes varicella zoster virus, Epstein-Barr virus, and cytomegalovirus. Like all herpesviruses, HSV tends to establish latent infection and eventually it reactivates and becomes infectious. Most HSV-infected patients have asymptomatic infections or the symptoms are only mildly uncomfortable. However, a substantial number of patients experience frequent painful recurrences or severe or life-threatening illnesses.

I. **Virology and pathogenesis**
- A. Two types of HSV exist: HSV-1 and HSV-2. Both types can infect any anatomic site.
- B. **HSV-1** may cause asymptomatic infection, oral lesions, nonoral or non-genital skin lesions, encephalitis, neonatal disease, and genital lesions
- C. **HSV-2** may cause asymptomatic infection, genital lesions, neonatal disease, nonoral, nongenital skin lesions, meningitis, and oral lesions

II. **Transmission**
- A. HSV-1 and HSV-2 are transmitted from person to person through contact with infected skin lesions, mucous membranes, and secretions. The incubation period is 1 to 26 days, and both types may be transmitted in utero or perinatally.
- B. Asymptomatic virus shedding may transmit the disease. Women who have had previous genital HSV-2 infection shed virus on 2% of days.
- C. **Oral/facial HSV infections**
  1. HSV-1 infection is extremely common in infants and children. The most common clinical manifestation of primary HSV-1 infection is gingivostomatitis, characterized by fever, malaise, myalgia, pharyngitis, irritability, and cervical adenopathy. The illness is self-limited and usually of short duration.
  2. Recurrent HSV-1 infections are most frequently characterized by oral and lip lesions. Many individuals who have oral HSV lesions have no known history of prior gingivostomatitis.
  3. HSV-2 also may cause oral lesions and pharyngitis, particularly in sexually active individuals.
- D. **Genital HSV infections**
  1. Many HSV infections are asymptomatic, but they can also cause papular, vesicular, or ulcerative lesions with pain, itching, urethral or vaginal discharge, and dysuria.
  2. Primary infections cause more severe symptoms and signs, including extensive skin lesions, tender inguinal adenopathy, and extragenital lesions. Primary infections are often associated with fever, headache, malaise, abdominal pain, and aseptic meningitis.
  3. Eighty percent of persons who have a first episode of HSV-2 genital infection will experience a recurrence in the first year. Most patients who have genital HSV infection have few symptomatic recurrences.

E. HSV encephalitis

1. HSV encephalitis is the most common viral infection of the CNS. The incidence peaks at 5 to 30 years and at more than 50 years. Ninety-five percent of cases are caused by HSV-1. HSV encephalitis is characterized by acute fever, altered mental status, and focal neurologic symptoms and signs.

2. Routine CSF findings are not diagnostic. Polymerase chain reaction (PCR) can detect HSV DNA in CSF. HSV is rarely isolated by culture of the CSF.

3. Electroencephalographic (EEG) findings can be diagnostic, with spike and slow wave activity localized to the temporal region.

4. CT scan and MRI may reveal localized edema and hemorrhage suggestive of HSV infection.

5. The prognosis for HSV encephalitis without treatment is poor, and even with antiviral therapy, substantial morbidity and mortality occurs. Prompt institution of empiric therapy is essential when the clinical diagnosis is suspected.

F. Neonatal HSV infections

1. Infection in neonates results from vertical transmission during the peripartum period in 85%; *in utero* or postpartum transmission rarely occurs. Seventy percent of untreated infants will progress to disseminated or CNS disease. Most neonatal infections are caused by HSV-2, although 30% of cases are caused by HSV-1. Seventy to 80% of infected infants are born to mothers who are unaware that they have genital HSV infection.

2. **Skin, eye, mouth (SEM) disease** accounts for 45% of peripartum infections. SEM disease most commonly presents in the first or second weeks of life with vesicular skin lesions which may occur anywhere on the body. Skin lesions have an erythematous base with clear or cloudy fluid. If the infection does not progress to involve the CNS or viscera, SEM disease has a low mortality.

3. **Central nervous system disease** is manifest as encephalitis, and it accounts for 35% of peripartum infections.

   a. Neonatal HSV CNS disease most commonly presents in the second to third week of life. Only 60% will develop skin lesions during the illness. HSV CNS disease has a 50% mortality if not treated; with treatment, mortality is 18%. The diagnosis must be considered in any infant who presents with encephalitis, seizures, apnea, bradycardia, or cranial nerve abnormalities.

   b. Cerebrospinal fluid findings are nonspecific and include pleocytosis and increased protein. Early initiation of therapy is critical when the diagnosis is suspected.

4. **Disseminated disease** is characterized by hepatitis, pneumonitis, and disseminated intravascular coagulation, and it accounts for 20% of peripartum infections.

   a. HSV disseminated disease presents in the first week of life. Bilateral patchy infiltrates are indicative of pneumonitis. Skin lesions may not be present initially.

   b. Disseminated HSV disease should be considered in any infant presenting with sepsis that is unresponsive to antibiotic therapy, or who has both pneumonitis and hepatitis.

5. **Eye infections**

   a. HSV is the most common cause of corneal blindness. HSV keratitis is characterized by conjunctivitis and dendritic lesions of the cornea.

   b. Topical steroids are contraindicated because they may facilitate spread of infection to the deep structures of the eyes.

III. Management of perinatal HSV infection

A. The most reliable predictor of the risk of perinatal transmission is whether a woman has active genital lesions at the time of delivery.

B. A thorough physical examination, including vaginal speculum exam, at the onset of labor should exclude the presence of active genital lesions. If HSV lesions are found during labor, prompt cesarean section is recommended.

C. Management of infants exposed to HSV at delivery

1. Virus cultures of the infant's conjunctivae, pharynx, skin folds, CSF, and rectum at 24-48 hours can indicate whether HSV has been transmitted. Infants who are culture positive for HSV from any site after 24 hours of life are given acyclovir.

2. During the time when HSV-exposed infants are in the hospital, they should be placed in contact isolation. Circumcision is deferred.

V. Diagnosis of HSV infection

A. HSV-1 and HSV-2 can be isolated by virus culture from active skin, eye, and genital lesions. In cases of recurrent disease, virus shedding may be too brief to be detected by virus culture. Herpes simplex is rarely is recovered from CSF by culture.

B. Although less sensitive and specific than culture, staining for virus antigens with fluorescent antibodies detects HSV more rapidly.

C. PCR is a useful diagnostic procedure for HSV encephalitis, with a sensitivity of 75% and a specificity of 100%.

VI. Therapy for HSV infections

A. Parenteral acyclovir is indicated for severe or potentially severe infections, such as neonatal HSV infection, HSV encephalitis, and non-localized infections in immunocompromised patients. Oral acyclovir decreases new lesion formation and improves symptoms in first episode genital HSV. Oral acyclovir has limited effect on the resolution of recurrent HSV disease.

B. Topical acyclovir is not effective for skin or oral lesions. The ophthalmic solution is useful for HSV keratitis, in combination with IV acyclovir.

C. Acyclovir (Zovirax)

1. For serious infections, such as neonatal disease and encephalitis, 5-10 mg/kg IV is given q8h for 10 to 21 days. Doses up to 20 mg/kg IV q8h are used for infants who have CNS or disseminated infection.

2. Oral acyclovir dosage is 20 mg/kg every 8 hours or 200 mg five times a day for 7-10 days. The adult regimen is 400 mg three times a day.

3. Suppression is indicated for immunocompromised patients or patients who have more than 6 genital recurrences a year; 5 mg/kg q8h or 400 mg bid. Suppressive therapy is also used for infants who have HSV SEM disease.

D. Valacyclovir (Valtrex) is an ester of acyclovir that has better oral absorption; 1 gm orally twice a day for 5 days. It has a more convenient dosage schedule than acyclovir and is approved for adolescents.

E. Famciclovir (Famvir) has a more convenient dosage schedule than acyclovir and is approved for adolescents. Dosage for first episodes of genital HSV infection is 250 mg q8h for 5 days, and for recurrent episodes it is 125 mg twice a day for 5 days.

F. Sexually active individuals known to have genital HSV infection should be advised to use latex condoms even during asymptomatic periods.

References, see page 164.

Urticaria, Angioedema and Anaphylaxis

Urticaria, angioedema, and anaphylaxis are manifestations of the immediate hypersensitivity reaction. Immediate hypersensitivity is an antibody mediated reaction that occurs within minutes to hours of exposure to a particular antigen by an immune individual. Twenty percent of the population will have one of these manifestations, especially urticaria, at some time during life.

I. Pathophysiology

A. **Urticaria** (or hives) is an intensely itchy rash that consists of raised, irregularly shaped wheals. The wheals have a blanched center, surrounded by a red flare. Antigens, chemicals and physical agents (detergents or ultraviolet light) can cause urticaria.

B. **Angioedema** is an area of circumscribed swelling of any part of the body. It may be caused by the same mechanisms that cause hives except that the immunologic events occur deeper in the cutis or in the submucosal tissue of the respiratory or gastrointestinal tract.

C. **Anaphylaxis** is the acute reaction that occurs when an antigen is introduced systemically into an individual who has preexisting IgE antibodies.

   1. The patient has difficulty breathing from constriction of the major airways and shock due to hypotension caused by histamine release.

   2. Anaphylactoid reactions are not immunologically mediated. Mannitol, radiocontrast material, and drugs (opiates, vancomycin) may degranulate mast cells and cause a reaction that resembles anaphylaxis.

II. Anaphylaxis

A. **Causes of anaphylaxis** include penicillins, insect venoms, airborne allergens, foods (peanuts, eggs, milk, seafoods, and food dyes and flavors), antitoxins to tetanus, and products of animal origin.

B. **Symptoms of anaphylaxis** include pruritus, injection of the mucous membranes, bronchospasm, and hypotension.

C. **Prevention of anaphylaxis.** Anaphylaxis is best prevented by avoidance of the cause. However, anaphylaxis frequently is unanticipated. Individuals with a history of anaphylaxis should be provided with injectable epinephrine. Short-term desensitization may be needed in a patient requiring antibiotic treatment.

D. **Treatment of acute anaphylaxis**

   1. Epinephrine in a 1:1000 dilution (1.0 mg/mL) should be injected at 10-20 min intervals at 0.01 mL/kg SQ per dose, with a maximum dose of 0.3 mL per dose SQ.

   2. Oxygen should be administered (100%, 4 L/min) and the airway should be secured.

   3. Albuterol, 0.1-0.2 mL/kg in a 5 mg/mL solution, should be given via nebulizer every 4-6 hours.

   4. Administration of diphenhydramine or chlorpheniramine and corticosteroids should be considered when a complete response to epinephrine does not occur.

III. Urticaria

A. **Hives** most commonly results from ingestion of foods, food additives, or drugs. These usually cause hive formation for only a few hours to two days.

B. **Cold urticaria** may be induced by exposure to cold, which may result in hypotension after immersion in cold water.

C. **Cholinergic urticaria** is characterized by the appearance of small punctate wheals, surrounded by a prominent erythematous flare. These small papular urtications are pruritic and appear predominantly on the neck and upper thorax. The lesions often develop after exercise, sweating, exposure to heat, or anxiety.

D. **Solar urticaria** may be caused by various wavelengths of light (280-500 nm). It is uncommon, and it is treated with sun screens.

E. **Chronic urticaria** is caused by ingestion of food substances that contain natural salicylates. Sensitivity to the food additive tartrazine yellow No. 5 frequently is found in patients with salicylate sensitivity.

F. **Exercise urticaria** is characterized by hives and bronchospasm after exercise.

G. **Genetic deficiencies of complement** factor H or factor I may cause urticaria. Patients who have these defects frequently develop severe hives, particularly after exposure to cold or hot water or alcohol ingestion.

H. Treatment of urticaria. Urticaria generally is a self-limiting disorder and usually requires only antihistamines. Hydroxyzine 0.5 mg/kg is the most effective treatment. Diphenhydramine 1.25 mg/kg every 6 hrs is also effective.

V. Angioedema

A. Angioedema is similar to hives, but the reaction occurs deeper in the dermis. It causes diffuse circumscribed swelling. Angioedema is often acquired, or it may be observed in an inherited disease known as hereditary angioneurotic edema (HANE).

B. Hereditary Angioneurotic Edema (HANE)

   1. HANE is characterized by episodes of localized subcutaneous edema of any part of the body. Attacks of severe abdominal cramps and vomiting may be caused by edema of the bowel wall. Severe attacks of colic may occur during infancy.

   2. Laryngeal edema may sometimes progress to total upper airway obstruction, pulmonary edema, and death. Attacks of palatal and laryngeal edema may follow dental trauma or occur during upper respiratory infections.

   3. HANE is inherited as an autosomal dominant disease. However, about 10% of cases are caused by new spontaneous mutations, which are passed to offspring.

   4. Prophylaxis against attacks of angioedema can be achieved with impeded androgens (ie, androgens that are only minimally virilizing). Stanozolol, at a dose of 2 mg/day; or danazol, 50-300 mg/day, can prevent attacks of angioedema.

C. Acute angioedema does not generally respond to epinephrine, antihistamines, or steroids. Treatment consists of supportive therapy with IV fluids, analgesics, and airway management. Fresh frozen plasma is generally effective.

References, see page 164.

Infectious Diseases

Fever Without Source in Infants and Young Children

Two-thirds of children visit their physician with an acute febrile illness before the age of three. The most common causes of fever in children are respiratory, urinary tract, gastrointestinal, and central nervous system infections. Bacteremia may occur with any of these infections.

I. **Clinical evaluation of the febrile child**. The child's health status, course of the current illness, birth and past medical history, and immunization should be evaluated. Infants at risk for serious bacterial infection include those with chronic illness, previous hospitalizations, prematurity, newborn complications, or previous antimicrobial therapy.

II. **Physical examination**
   A. Fever is defined as a rectal temperature of at least 38.0°C (100.4°F). Axillary and tympanic measurements are unreliable.
   B. **Toxicity** is characterized by signs of sepsis (lethargy, poor perfusion, marked hypoventilation or hyperventilation, or cyanosis). The quality of cry, reaction to parents, color, state of hydration, response to social overtures, affect, respiratory status and effort, and peripheral perfusion should be assessed.

Clinical and Laboratory Findings in Toxic and Non-toxic Infants and Children

Febrile Infants at Low Risk	Toxic Infant or Child

History
   No previous hospitalizations or chronic illness
   Term delivery without complications
   No previous antibiotic therapy
Physical Examination
   Nontoxic clinical appearance
   No focal bacterial infection (except otitis media)
   Activity, hydration and perfusion normal
Social Situation
   Parents/caregiver mature and reliable
   Thermometer and telephone at child's home
Laboratory Criteria
   White blood cell count of 5,000-15,000/mm³
   Band cell count <1,500/mm³
   Normal urinalysis (<5 white blood cells/high-power field)
   When diarrhea is present, less than 5 white blood cells/high-power field in stool
	Slow, irregular or decreasing respiratory rate
	Head bobbing
	Stridor
	Paradoxic or abdominal breathing
	Chest retractions
	Central cyanosis
	Altered level of consciousness
	Fever with petechiae
	Tachypnea
	Grunting
	Prolonged expiration
	Nasal flaring
	Poor muscle tone
	Poor or delayed capillary refill
	Tachycardia

   C. Neonates with acute bacterial meningitis often lack meningismus. Meningitis in neonates may manifest as temperature instability (hyperthermia or hypothermia), poor feeding, listlessness, lethargy, irritability, vomiting, or respiratory distress.

A bulging fontanelle may be seen in one-third of cases.

D. In older infants and children, initial symptoms of bacterial meningitis consist of fever, signs of increased intracranial pressure, and cerebral cortical dysfunction. Fever in children who have bacterial meningitis usually is greater than 38.3°C.

E. Older children and adolescents frequently present with headache, fever, altered sensorium, and meningismus. Kernig's or Brudzinski's signs may be absent in up to 50% of adolescents and adults with meningitis.

III. Laboratory studies

A. Reassuring laboratory screening values include a white blood cell count of 5,000 to 15,000/mm³ (5.0 to 15.0 x 10/L), an absolute band cell count of <1,500/mm³, and fewer than 5 white blood cells per high-power field in stool specimens in infants with diarrhea.

B. **Gram-stained smear of urine sediment** is a sensitive screening test; a urine culture should be obtained to confirm urinary tract infection.

C. **Blood cultures** are valuable in confirming bacteremia.

D. **Lumbar puncture** is mandatory when the diagnosis of meningitis is suspected in a febrile child.

IV. Management of fever without source

A. **Toxic-appearing infants and children.** All toxic-appearing febrile infants and children less than 36 months of age should be hospitalized for evaluation and treatment of meningitis or possible sepsis.

B. **Febrile infants less than 28 days of age**
   1. Fever in infants less than 28 days of age mandates a sepsis evaluation and hospitalization for parenteral antibiotic therapy until culture results are known.
   2. Laboratory evaluation includes an examination of cerebrospinal fluid for cells, glucose, protein and culture; a urinalysis and urine culture; and a blood culture.

C. **Febrile infants 28 to 90 days of age**
   1. Infants who do not meet low-risk criteria should be hospitalized for a sepsis evaluation and empiric antimicrobial therapy until culture results are known.
   2. Febrile infants less than three months of age who meet low-risk criteria, can be observed after a urine culture has been obtained.
   3. Empiric parenteral antimicrobial therapy may be used in the outpatient management of low-risk infants. Ceftriaxone (Rocephin), a third-generation parenteral cephalosporin with a half-life of 5-6 hours, is often used; 50 mg/kg IM qd.
   4. Children who have met low-risk criteria with reliable parents can be treated as outpatients if close follow-up within 18-24 hours can be ensured. Caregivers are instructed to check the child every 4 hours for activity, rectal temperature, and skin color.

D. **Febrile children 3 months to 36 months of age**
   1. Occult bacteremia in febrile children 3 to 36 months of age without a source of infection has an incidence of 3-11%, with a mean probability of 4.3% in children with a temperature of at least 39.0°C (102.2°F).
   2. Nontoxic-appearing children with a fever of less than 39.0°C (102.2°F), who have been previously healthy, may be managed expectantly if there is no apparent focus of infection. Acetaminophen, 15 mg/kg/dose q4h, is given for fever, and the child is reevaluated if the fever persists for more than 48 hours or if the child's clinical condition worsens.
   3. Children with a fever greater than 39.0°C (102.2°F) may require a lumbar puncture, white blood cell count, and empiric antimicrobial therapy.
      a. Children with a white blood cell count of 15,000/mm³ or more require a blood culture and treatment with empiric antimicrobial therapy.
      b. Children with a white blood cell count of less than 15,000/mm³ and a benign clinical appearance can be managed expectantly with antipyretics and

return of the child if fever persists for more than 48 hours or if the child's clinical condition worsens.

References, see page 164.

Bacterial Meningitis

Bacterial meningitis affects 1 in 500 children younger than 2 years. Meningitis most commonly presents with subtle signs and symptoms

I. **Etiology of Bacterial Meningitis**
   A. **Neonatal Meningitis – 0 to 3 Months of Age**
      1. The most common bacterial agents responsible for CNS infection in infants 0 to 3 months of life (in declining order of frequency) are: group B *Streptococcus* (GBS), *Escherichia coli*, *Listeria*, *Enterococcus*, Gram-negative enteric bacilli other than *E coli*, fungi, and anaerobes.
      2. The preterm infant is considered an immunocompromised host; thus, all agents should be considered, including bacteria, viruses, *Mycoplasma*, *Ureaplasma*, and fungi, as potential causes of CNS infection in this group.

Common Etiologic Agents of Meningitis by Age Group				
Organism	0-3 Months	3-36 Months	3-21 Years	Immuno-compromised
Group B Streptococcus	X			
Escherichia coli	X			
Listeria monocytogenes	X			
Streptococcus pneumoniae		X	X	X
Neisseria meningitidis		X	X	X
Fungus				X
Cryptococcus				X
Tuberculosis		X		
Virus	X	X	X	X

Note: Haemophilus influenzae no longer is a common pathogen in countries where the conjugate vaccines are used routinely.

   B. **Infancy – 3 Months to 3 Years**. Since the advent of the *Haemophilus* conjugate vaccines, the principal causes of bacterial meningitis in this age group are *N meningitidis* and *S pneumoniae*.

C. **Childhood – 3 to 21 Years**. The most common bacterial agents for meningitis in this age group are *N meningitidis* and *S pneumoniae*. Viral meningitis, principally caused by the enteroviruses, arboviruses and herpesviruses, account for most of the CNS disease in this age group.

I. **Clinical evaluation**
  A. **Signs and symptoms** of meningitis include fever, headache, neck pain or stiffness, nausea, vomiting, photophobia, and irritability. Young infants may exhibit only signs of irritability, somnolence, and low-grade fever.
  B. **Physical findings** include lethargy, somnolence, stiff neck, rash, petechia, purpura, and hemodynamic instability.
  C. **Lumbar puncture** remains the most important early diagnostic test.
     1. **Rapid antigen testing** of the CSF and urine are specific but not sensitive indicators of disease; with the exception of Haemophilus meningitis, it rarely provides helpful information in guiding initial therapy.
     2. **Gram stain of a CSF smear** is very helpful. CSF protein levels greater than 100 to 120 mg/dL are suggestive of bacterial meningitis, but these also can be seen in congenital infection, tuberculous meningitis, and rarely, in viral CNS disease.
     3. **Culture.** The standard for diagnosis of meningitis remains a positive culture taken before initiation of antibiotic therapy.
     4. **Blood culture**, Gram stain of a CSF smear, CSF culture, urinalysis, and urine culture should be performed routinely in all children who are suspected clinically of having meningitis. If the CSF indices suggest viral, fungal, or tuberculous disease, specific stains and cultures should be requested.
     5. **CSF analysis** must include cell count, differential, and protein and glucose concentrations.
  D. When viral meningitis is suspected, rectal swabs, CSF and peripheral buffy coat viral cultures, and PCR should be considered. Isolation of virus from any site suggests the possibility of viral meningitis if the CSF indices are abnormal, but coinfection with bacteria can occur. For the immunocompromised patient, cryptococcal antigen or an India ink-stained smear of CSF provides quick identification.
  E. Complete blood count, platelet count, and serum electrolyte concentrations are helpful as baseline studies. Liver enzymes can be greatly elevated with enterovirus and disseminated herpetic infection.

Cerebrospinal Fluid Findings in Normal and Infected Hosts					
Disorder	Color	WBC Count ($/mm^3$)	Glucose (mg/dL)	Protein (mg/dL)	Gram's Stain and culture
Normal infant	clear	<10	>40	90	negative
Normal child or adult	clear	0	>40	<40	negative
Bacterial meningitis	cloudy	200-10000	<40	100-500	usually positive
Viral meningitis	clear	25-1000 (<50% PMN)	>40	50-100	negative

III. Management of bacterial meningitis

A. **Term infants in the first month of life** are treated with a combination of ampicillin with either gentamicin or cefotaxime. For low-birthweight preterm infants in the nursery who present with late-onset meningitis, an antistaphylococcal agent such as methicillin or vancomycin and an aminoglycoside are used until culture results are available.

B. **Infants 1 to 2 months of age** are treated with ampicillin and cefotaxime or ampicillin and ceftriaxone, which provide coverage against enterococci and *Listeria* as well as the normal pathogens beyond the newborn period.

C. **Infants and children older than 2 months of age.** Resistant strains of *S pneumoniae* have become a major problem. Initial meningitis therapy must include vancomycin in dosages of 60 mg/kg per day in four divided doses in addition to either cefotaxime or ceftriaxone. This dosage of vancomycin should be adjusted to maintain peak serum concentrations of 30 to 40 mcg/mL and trough values of 5 to 10 mcg/mL. The initial dosage of cefotaxime (Claforan) is 75 mg/kg per dose every 6 hours. Ceftriaxone (Rocephin) dosage is 80 to 100 mg/kg daily in one dose; an extra dose is given on the first day at 12 hours.

Dosages of Antibiotics Administered Intravenously to Newborn Infants and Children

Antibiotic	Age (Days)	Dosage	Desired Serum Concentrations (Mcg/mL)
Ampicillin	0-7 7-30 >30	50 mg/kg/dose q8h 50-75 mg/kg/dose q6h 50-75 q6h	Not critical to measure
Cefotaxime (Claforan)	0-7 7-30 >30	50 mg/kg/dose q8h 50-75 mg/kg/dose q6h 75 q6h	Not critical to measure
Ceftriaxone (Rocephin)	All	80-100 mg/kg/dose. At diagnosis, 12 h, 24 h, and every 24 h thereafter	Not critical to measure
Gentamicin	0-7 7-30 >30	2.5 mg/kg/dose q12h 2.5 mg/kg/dose q8h 2.5 mg/kg/dose q8h	Peak, 6-10 Trough,<2
Vancomycin	0-7 7-30 >30	15 mg/kg/dose q12h 15 mg/kg/dose q8h 15 mg/kg/dose q6h	Peak, 30-40 Trough, 5-10

D. **Dexamethasone.** If CSF indices suggest bacterial meningitis or if organisms are seen on Gram stain of a CSF smear, dexamethasone is recommended in a dosage of 0.6 mg/kg per day in two to four divided doses for 2 to 4 days. The initial dose of steroid should be infused before the initial dose of parenteral antibiotics.

References, see page 164.

Otitis Media

Otitis media is the most commonly diagnosed illness in childhood. This infection occurs in half of all infants before their first birthday and in 80% by their third birthday. Half of all infected children will have 3 or more episodes in their first 3 years of life.

I. Pathophysiology

A. **Acute otitis media** consists of inflammation of the middle ear. Fever and ear pain are the most common acute symptoms. Irritability, anorexia, vomiting, and diarrhea may also be present. Acute otitis media is most common in children 6 months to 3 years. The majority of children have had at least one episode of acute otitis by age 3. It is uncommon after age 8. The incidence rises during winter and declines during summer.

B. **Otitis media with effusion** consists of a chronic bacterial infection persisting more than 2 weeks, manifesting as an asymptomatic middle-ear effusion. The syndrome usually develops after an acute otitis media.

II. Microbiology

A. **Common pathogens.** The most common bacterial pathogen in all age groups is Streptococcus pneumoniae, causing 40% of effusions. The next most common is non-typable Haemophilus influenzae, causing 20% of effusions. Anaerobic bacteria, Chlamydia or Mycoplasma cause less than 2-5%.

B. **Ampicillin resistence** caused by beta-lactamase occurs in 30-50% of H influenzae and up to 80% of M. catarrhalis.

C. **Penicillin-resistant S. pneumoniae** results from bacterial alterations in penicillin-binding proteins, rather than beta-lactamase. Highly resistant strains are resistant to penicillin, trimethoprim/sulfamethoxazole (TMP/SMX), and third-generation cephalosporins. The prevalence of multiple-drug resistant S. pneumoniae is 20-35%.

III. Diagnosis

A. **Acute otitis media**

1. The position, color, translucency and mobility of the tympanic membrane should be assessed. The normal eardrum is translucent, and landmarks should be visible through the eardrum. A cloudy opacified tympanic membrane in children is often associated with a middle-ear effusion. Erythema of the eardrum alone is often the result of a viral infection or crying.

2. In otitis media, the tympanic membrane is dull and bulges externally, losing its concave contour and light reflex. An air-fluid level or air bubbles may sometimes be visualized behind the tympanic membrane.

3. Reduced or absent mobility of the tympanic membrane with air insufflation is the most specific sign of acute otitis media.

B. **Otitis media with effusion.** In the absence of symptoms or signs of acute illness, evidence of middle- ear inflammation indicates that an otitis media with effusion is present. Typical findings include diminished tympanic membrane mobility and visualization of air-fluid levels.

IV. Treatment of acute otitis media

A. **First-line antibiotics**

1. Oral antibiotics should be prescribed for 10-14 days.

2. **Amoxicillin** is the first-line antimicrobial agent for treating AOM, at doses of 80-90 mg/kg/d. For patients with treatment failure after three days of therapy, alternative agents include oral amoxicillin-clavulanate, cefuroxime axetil, and intramuscular ceftriaxone.

3. **Streptococcus pneumoniae** causes 40-50% of all cases of AOM. This bacterium has reduced susceptibility to penicillin in 8-35% (2-4% highly resistant) of isolates and reduced susceptibility to third-generation cephalosporins in 10% of isolates

(about 4% highly resistant).

4. **Cefuroxime axetil (Ceftin) and amoxicillin-clavulanate (Augmentin) orally, and ceftriaxone (Rocephin) intramuscularly,** are useful as second-line drugs for treatment failure after three days of therapy.

Second-Line Antibiotic Therapy for Acute Otitis Media		
Drug	Dosage	Comments
Amoxicillin-clavulanic acid (Augmentin)	40 mg/kg of amoxicillin component in 3 divided doses	Diarrhea common
Cefuroxime axetil (Ceftin)	500 mg in 2 divided doses	
Ceftriaxone (Rocephin)	50 mg/kg IM	

References, see page 164.

Pneumonia

A lower respiratory tract infection (LRI) develops in one in three children in the first year of life. Twenty-nine percent of these children develop pneumonia, 15% develop croup, 34% tracheobronchitis, and 29% bronchiolitis.

I. **Clinical evaluation of pneumonia**
   A. **Cough**. Pneumonia usually causes cough that persists day and night. Patients who cough spontaneously throughout the office visit are likely to have lower respiratory tract disease.
   B. **Grunting** occurs in 20% of infants who have bronchiolitis or pneumonia. Grunting prevents collapse of narrowed airways and improves oxygenation.
   C. **Chest pain**. Pneumonia causes chest pain when the infection develops near the pleura. Pneumonia that involves the diaphragmatic pleura may present as abdominal pain. Older children may complain of diffuse chest or abdominal pain, which is caused by persistent cough and repeated muscle contraction.
   D. **Tachypnea**. Increased respiratory rate is one of the earliest and most consistent signs of lower respiratory tract disease.

Abnormal Respiratory Rates by Age	
Age	Abnormal
<2 months	>60 bpm
2-12 months old	>50 bpm
>1 year old	>40 bpm

   E. **Retractions**. Retractions of the intercostal spaces may occur with pneumonia because of decreased compliance or increased airway resistance.
   F. **Auscultation**
      1. **Signs of consolidation** include dullness to percussion and increased transmission

of the voice on auscultation.

2. **Crackles** are the fine popping sounds that occur when previously closed airways open suddenly. They indicate pulmonary parenchymal disease.

3. **Wheezing** is generated by narrowed airways. It can be caused by bronchiolitis, asthma, early pulmonary edema, subglottic stenosis, or tracheal compression.

G. **Cyanosis** occurs at an oxygen saturation of 67%; however, cyanosis will not manifest in the presence of anemia. It is not a sensitive predictor of pneumonia because significant hypoxemia may be present before cyanosis is visible.

II. Diagnostic evaluation of lower respiratory infections

A. **Chest radiograph.** A chest radiograph should be obtained when the child with pneumonia appears acutely ill.

B. **Laboratory tests**

1. **WBC count** should be obtained for children who have significant fever (>38°C in infants, >39°C in children), who appear ill, or who are hospitalized.

2. **Blood cultures** are rarely positive in children with pneumonia. They should be obtained in infants and children with high fever, ill appearance, or upon hospitalization.

3. **Bacterial antigen assays** of urine by latex agglutination, or antibody tests of blood are indicated when unusual infections are suspected or when pneumonia is unresponsive to therapy.

4. **Nasopharyngeal cultures for viruses** and immunofluorescence studies for viral antigens are obtained when therapy with antiviral agents is being considered.

III. Pneumonia in newborns

A. **Group B streptococcal disease** is the most common cause of pneumonia in the newborn. The infection usually is acquired in utero. Prenatal screening of expectant mothers and intrapartum prophylaxis of colonized mothers with IV ampicillin has decreased the incidence.

B. Initial therapy of pneumonia in newborns consists of ampicillin (100 mg/kg IV initial dose, followed by 200 mg/kg/day divided QID) and gentamicin (2.5 mg/kg IV initial dose, followed by 7.5 mg/kg/day divided q8h).

IV. Neonates

A. Bacterial pneumonia in the first day of life may be impossible to distinguish from hyaline membrane disease or transient tachypnea of the newborn. Therefore, respiratory distress in newborns should be treated as bacterial pneumonia until proven otherwise. When associated with chorioamnionitis, it is caused most commonly by Escherichia coli or by group B streptococci (GBS). However, Haemophilus influenzae, Streptococcus pneumoniae (pneumococcus), group D streptococci, Listeria, and anaerobes also may be present in this setting.

B. Infants also may develop bacterial pneumonia transnatally, secondary to GBS. The onset of symptoms tends to occur 12 to 24 hours after birth.

C. Chest radiographs of infants who have bacterial pneumonia may exhibit a diffuse reticular nodular appearance, but, in contrast to hyaline membrane disease, they tend to show normal or increased lung volumes with possible focal or coarse densities.

D. In the newborn who has bacterial pneumonia, blood cultures obtained before the initiation of antibiotics commonly grow the offending organism. Cultures of urine and cerebrospinal fluid should be obtained at the time of the blood culture.

E. **Empiric treatment** should be initiated with ampicillin 100 mg/kg per day divided every 12 hours (infants <1.2 kg) or every 8 hours (infants >1.2 kg) and cefotaxime 100 mg/kg per day divided every 12 hours or 150 mg/kg per day divided every 8 hours (infants >1.2 kg and >7 d old). Gentamicin is an alternative. Treatment should be continued for at least 10 days.

V. Infants

- **A.** In the infant who is younger than 6 months of age, pneumonia is characterized by fever of abrupt onset (generally >38.5°C [101.3°F]) and a productive-sounding cough. There may be signs of systemic toxicity (decreased peripheral perfusion with delayed capillary refill, lethargy, tachycardia).
- **B.** Tachypnea (respiratory rate >50 breaths/min at rest) is the most sensitive sign of pneumonia in infants. Infants who have bacterial pneumonia often have retractions, and they may have auscultatory evidence of lung disease. Cyanosis, nasal flaring, and expiratory grunting are suggestive of a severe pneumonia in infants.
- **C.** Pneumococcus is the most common cause of bacterial pneumonia in infants. Other common organisms include S aureus, Moraxella catarrhalis, and H influenzae. H influenzae type b (Hib) is an uncommon cause because of Hib vaccine.
- **D.** Infants in whom bacterial pneumonia is suspected require blood and urine cultures and a complete blood count. Cerebrospinal culture analysis is advisable in ill-appearing infants, particularly those younger than 3 months of age.
- **E.** **Chest radiography.** Focal consolidation is characteristic of bacterial pneumonia.
- **F.** Oxygen therapy and fluid resuscitation should be undertaken.
- **G.** The infant suspected of having bacterial pneumonia should be treated with parenteral ampicillin/sulbactam (Unasyn), given as 200 mg/kg per 24 hours divided every 6 hours. Cefuroxime (Zinacef) (150 mg/kg per 24 hours divided every 8 hours) or ceftriaxone (Rocephin) (75 mg/kg per 24 hours divided every 12 to 24 hours) are reasonable alternatives. Once the infant has defervesced and is stable, he can be switched to amoxicillin/clavulanic acid (Augmentin) (40 mg/kg per day divided every 8 hours) to complete a 10-day course.

VI. Preschool-age children

- **A.** Pneumococcus is the most common cause of bacterial pneumonia in preschool-age children. Moraxella, Hib, and Neisseria meningitidis each cause a small fraction of bacterial pneumonias.
- **B.** The febrile, tachypneic (>40 breaths/min) child who has a cough should have a chest radiograph. Radiography likely will reveal a lobar or segmental consolidation. Rounded, circular-appearing infiltrates are common in bacterial pneumonia at this age. A complete blood count and blood culture should be obtained for children younger than 2 years.
- **C.** Children who are hypoxemic, in respiratory distress, or hemodynamically unstable should be admitted to the hospital and treated with parenteral ampicillin/sulbactam (Unasyn) (200 mg/kg per 24 hours divided every 6 hours) or cefuroxime (Zinacef) (150 mg/kg per 24 hours divided every 8 hours) until the patient is more stable and can be switched to amoxicillin/clavulanic acid (Augmentin)(40 mg/kg per day divided every 8 hours).
- **D.** Patients who are not hypoxemic, in distress, or unstable and who have reliable caretakers at home can be treated with amoxicillin/clavulanic acid (Augmentin) 40 mg/kg per day divided every 8 hours for 10 days as an outpatient, although an initial dose of parenteral antibiotic may be of benefit. Macrolide antibiotics, particularly azithromycin [(Zithromax) 10 mg/kg (max 500 mg) PO on day 1 followed by 5 mg/kg on days 2-5] and clarithromycin [(Biaxin) 15 mg/kg/day PO bid), may be of some advantage if mycoplasma pneumoniae is suspected or if the patient is living in an area that has a high prevalence of penicillin-insensitive pneumococcus.
- **E.** The majority of pneumonia in preschool children is caused by RSV, influenza, parainfluenza, adenovirus, picornaviruses, and Mycoplasma. Patients who have nonbacterial pneumonia present with cough and wheezes or crackles. These patients are not toxic or in distress.

VII. School-age children/adolescents

- **A.** Mycoplasma and C pneumoniae (TWAR) are substantially more important pathogens in this population. Approximately 1 in 1,000 children between 10 and 15 years of age develop Mycoplasma pneumonia. However, bacteria, particularly pneumococcus, continue to be important pathogens.

B. **Physical examination.** Pulmonary consolidation is characterized by rales, dullness to percussion, increased tactile fremitus (eg, to the word "99") and increased whispered pectoriloquy (transmission of whispered syllables on auscultation).

C. Bacterial pneumonia is characterized by abrupt onset of high fever and cough productive of thick sputum that is rust-colored or bloody. Adolescents and some older children may be able to produce sputum for Gram stain and culture.

D. **Treatment** consists of ampicillin (100 mg/kg per day IV divided every 6 hours) for patients who are hypoxic or severely ill. If there is substantial concern about resistance or about the patient's clinical status, ceftriaxone (80 mg/kg per day once daily or divided twice daily) or a macrolide can be used. Parenteral ampicillin/sulbactam (Unasyn) (200 mg/kg per 24 hours divided every 6 hours) or cefuroxime (Zinacef) (150 mg/kg per 24 hours divided every 8 hours) or oral ampicillin/clavulanic acid (40 mg/kg per day divided every 8 hours) can be used if the sputum Gram stain suggests that H influenzae or S aureus is the causative organism.

E. Viruses, Mycoplasma, and C pneumoniae (TWAR) account for the majority of cases of pneumonia in adolescents. Mycoplasma infection often begins with the prodrome of headache or gastrointestinal symptoms as well as a low-grade fever. Rhinorrhea is not common. The cough frequently is productive, but the sputum is scant and nonbloody. The patient may have an erythematous macular rash or urticaria.

F. The older child and adolescent who has clinical evidence of Mycoplasma or TWAR pneumonia should be treated with a macrolide antibiotic or a tetracycline. Azithromycin (Zithromax) 500 mg on day 1, followed by 250 mg/d for four subsequent days is commonly used. Erythromycin or tetracycline (for children older than 8 years of age) is an alternative.

References, see page 164.

Bronchiolitis

Bronchiolitis is an acute wheezing-associated illness, which occurs in early life, preceded by signs and symptoms of an upper respiratory infection. Infants may have a single episode or may have multiple occurrences in the first year of life.

I. **Epidemiology**
   A. Bronchiolitis occurs most frequently from early November and continues through April.
   B. Bronchiolitis is most serious in infants who are less than one year old, especially those 1-3 months old. Infants at risk include those who are raised in crowded living conditions, who are passively exposed to tobacco smoke, and who are not breast-fed.

II. **Pathophysiology**
   A. Respiratory syncytial virus (RSV) is the leading cause of bronchiolitis in infants and young children, accounting for 50% of cases of bronchiolitis requiring hospitalization.
   B. Infants born prematurely, or with chronic lung disease (CLD), immunodeficiency or congenital heart disease are at especially high risk for severe RSV illness.
   C. RSV is transmitted by contact with nasal secretions. Shedding of virus occurs 1 to 2 days before symptoms occur, and for 1 to 2 weeks afterwards. Symptoms usually last an average of 5 days.
   D. Parainfluenza viruses are the second most frequent cause of bronchiolitis. They

cause illness during autumn and spring, before and after outbreaks of RSV. Influenza A virus, adenovirus, rhinovirus and Mycoplasma pneumonia can all cause bronchiolitis. Rhinovirus and mycoplasma pneumonia cause wheezing-associated respiratory illness in older children, while parainfluenza virus and RSV can cause wheezing at any age.

III. Clinical evaluation of bronchiolitis

A. Symptoms of RSV may range from those of a mild cold to severe bronchiolitis or pneumonia. RSV infection frequently begins with nasal discharge, pharyngitis, and cough. Hoarseness or laryngitis is not common. Fever occurs in most young children, with temperatures ranging from 38°°C to 40°°C (100.4°°F to 104°°F).

B. **Hyperresonance of the chest wall** may be present, and wheezing can be heard in most infants without auscultation. The wheezing sound is harsh and low in pitch, although severely affected infants may not have detectable wheezing. Fine "crackles" are usually heard on inspiration. Substernal and intercostal retractions are often noted.

C. **Cyanosis** of the oral mucosa and nail beds may occur in severely ill infants. Restlessness and hyperinflation of the chest wall are signs of impending respiratory failure.

IV. Diagnosis

A. Infants with bronchiolitis present symptoms of an upper respiratory illness for several days and wheezing during the peak RSV season.

B. **Chest radiography** typically shows hyperexpansion and diffuse interstitial pneumonitis. Consolidation is noted in about 25% of children, most commonly in the right upper or middle lobe.

C. **Oxygen saturation** values of <95% suggest the need for hospitalization.

D. **Arterial blood gases** should be obtained to assess the severity of respiratory compromise. Carbon dioxide levels are commonly in the 30-35 mm Hg range. Respiratory failure is suggested by CO_2 values of 45-55 mm Hg. Oxygen tension below 66 mm Hg indicates severe disease.

E. **White blood cell count** may be normal or elevated slightly, and the differential count may show neutrophilia.

F. **Enzyme-linked immunosorbent assays** (ELISA) of nasal washings for RSV are highly sensitive and specific.

V. Management

A. Outpatient management of bronchiolitis is appropriate for infants with mild disease.

B. **Criteria for hospitalization**
1. History of prematurity (especially less than 34 weeks)
2. Congenital heart disease
3. Other underlying lung disease
4. Low initial oxygen saturation suggestive of respiratory failure (O_2 saturation <95%, with a toxic, distressed appearance)
5. Age ≤3 months
6. Dehydrated infant who is not feeding well
7. Unreliable parents

C. Before hospitalization, infants should receive an aerosolized beta-adrenergic agent. A few infants will respond to this therapy and avoid hospitalization. If the response is good, the infant can be sent home, and oral albuterol continued.

D. Hospitalized infants should receive hydration and ambient oxygen to maintain an oxygen saturation ≥92-93% by pulse oximetry.

E. **Treatment of bronchiolitis in the hospital**
1. **Racemic epinephrine by inhalation** may be administered as a therapeutic trial. It should be continued if an improvement in the respiratory status is noted. Racemic epinephrine is administered as 0.5 mL of a 2.25% solution, diluted with 3.5 mL of saline (1:8) by nebulization. It is given every 20-30 minutes for

severe croup, and it is given every 4-6 hours for moderate croup.

2. **Ribavirin,** an antiviral agent, produces modest improvement in clinical illness and oxygenation. Ribavirin is helpful in severely ill or high-risk patients. The dosage is 2 gm (diluted to 60 mg/mL) aerosolized over 2 hours tid for 3-5 days using an oxygen hood. Treatment with ribavirin combined with RSV immune globulin administered either parenterally or by aerosol is more effective than therapy with either agent alone. Corticosteroid use in the treatment of bronchiolitis is not recommended.

Indications for Ribavirin Use in Bronchiolitis

Congenital heart disease, especially cyanotic	Immunodeficiency due to chemotherapy
	Cystic fibrosis
Chronic lung disease	Severe combined immunodeficiency
Renal transplantation, recent	Multiple congenital anomalies
Age <6 weeks	Certain premature infants
Neurologic diseases	Metabolic diseases
Heart failure of any cause	RSV bronchiolitis and a rising pCO_2
RSV bronchiolitis and arterial O_2 <65 mmHg	

VI. **Prevention of RSV Infections**
   A. Palivizumab (Synagis) is a humanized mouse monoclonal antibody that is given intramuscularly. Palivizumab is administered intramuscularly in a dose of 15 mg/kg once a month during the RSV season.

Recommendations by the American Academy of Pediatrics for the use of palivizumab (Synagis) and RSV-IGIV:

- Palivizumab (Synagis) or RSV-IGIV prophylaxis should be considered for infants and children younger than 2 years of age with chronic lung disease (CLD) who have required medical therapy for CLD within 6 months before the anticipated RSV season. Palivizumab is preferred for most high-risk children because of its ease of administration, safety, and effectiveness. Patients with more severe CLD may benefit from prophylaxis for 2 RSV seasons, especially those who require medical therapy.
- Infants born at 32 weeks of gestation or earlier without CLD or who do not meet the aforementioned criteria also may benefit from RSV prophylaxis. Infants born at 28 weeks of gestation or earlier may benefit from prophylaxis up to 12 months of age. Infants born at 29 to 32 weeks of gestation may benefit most from prophylaxis up to 6 months of age. Decisions about duration of prophylaxis should be individualized according to the duration of the RSV season.
- For patients born between 32 and 35 weeks of gestation, the use of palivizumab and RSV IGIV should be reserved for infants with additional risk factors.
- Prophylaxis for RSV should be initiated at the onset of the RSV season and terminated at the end of the RSV season. In most areas of the United States, the usual time for the beginning of RSV outbreaks is October to December, and termination is March to May, but regional differences occur.
- Palivizumab does not interfere with the response to vaccines.

References, see page 164.

Pharyngitis

Approximately 30 to 65 percent of pharyngitis cases are idiopathic, and 30 to 60 percent have a viral etiology (rhinovirus, adenovirus). Only 5 to 10 percent of sore throats are caused by bacteria, with group A beta-hemolytic streptococci being the most common. Other bacteria that occasionally cause pharyngitis include groups C and G streptococci, *Neisseria gonorrhoeae*, *Mycoplasma pneumoniae*, *Chlamydia pneumoniae*, and *Arcanobacterium haemolyticus*.

I. Clinical presentation

A. Pharyngitis caused by group A beta-hemolytic streptococci has an incubation period of two to five days and is most common in children five to 12 years of age. The illness is diagnosed most often in the winter and spring.

B. Group A beta-hemolytic streptococcal pharyngitis usually is an acute illness with sore throat and a temperature higher than 38.5°C (101.3°F). Constitutional symptoms include fever and chills, myalgias, headaches and nausea. Physical findings may include petechiae of the palate, pharyngeal and tonsillar erythema and exudates, and anterior cervical adenopathy.

C. Patients with cough or coryza, are less likely to have streptococcal pharyngitis. A sandpaper-like rash on the trunk, which is sometimes linear on the groin and axilla (Pastia's lines), is consistent with scarlet fever.

Features of Streptococcal Tonsillopharyngitis

Sudden onset	Marked inflammation of throat and tonsils
Sore throat (pain on swallowing)	Patchy discrete exudate
Fever	Tender, enlarged anterior cervical nodes
Headache	Scarlet fever
Nausea, vomiting, abdominal pain (especially in children)	

Features rarely associated with streptococcal tonsillopharyngitis–suggestive of other etiologies

Conjunctivitis	Diarrhea
Cough	Nasal discharge (except in young children)
Laryngitis (stridor, croup)	Muscle aches/malaise

II. Diagnostic Testing

A. Throat culture is the gold standard for the diagnosis of streptococcal pharyngitis. The sensitivity of throat culture for group A beta-hemolytic streptococci is 90 percent. The specificity of throat culture is 99 percent.

B. A rapid antigen detection test (rapid strep test) can be completed in five to 10 minutes. This test has a specificity of greater than 95 percent but a sensitivity of only 76 to 87 percent.

C. A positive rapid antigen detection test may be considered definitive evidence for treatment of streptococcal pharyngitis. A confirmatory throat culture should follow a negative rapid antigen detection test when the diagnosis of group A beta-hemolytic streptococcal infection is strongly suspected.

Complications of Group A Beta-Hemolytic Streptococcal Pharyngitis

Nonsuppurative complications

Rheumatic fever
Poststreptococcal glomerulonephritis

Suppurative complications

Cervical lymphadenitis	Otitis media
Peritonsillar or retropharyngeal abscess	Meningitis
	Bacteremia
Sinusitis	Endocarditis
Mastoiditis	Pneumonia

D. The annual incidence of acute rheumatic fever is one case per 1 million population. Suppurative complications of streptococcal pharyngitis occur as infection spreads from pharyngeal mucosa to deeper tissues.

II. Antibiotic Therapy

Selected Antibiotic Regimens for Group A Beta-Hemolytic Streptococcal Pharyngitis

Antibiotic	Dose/dosage	Dosing frequency	Duration
Penicillin V (Veetids)	Child: 250 mg	Two or three times daily	10 days
	Adult: 500 mg	Two or three times daily	10 days
Penicillin G benzathine (Bicillin L-A)	Child: 600,000 units	Single injection	--
	Adult: 1,200,000 units	Single injection	--
Amoxicillin (Amoxil)	Child: 40 mg per kg per day	Three divided doses	10 days
	Adult: 500 mg	Three times daily	10 days
Erythromycin ethylsuccinate (E.E.S. 400)	Child: 40 mg per kg per day	Two to four divided doses	10 days
	Adult: 400 mg	Four times daily	10 days
Erythromycin estolate	Child: 20 to 40 mg per kg per day	Two to four divided doses	10 days
	Adult: not recommended	--	--

Azithromycin (Zithromax)	Child: 10 mg per kg on day 1; 5 mg per kg on days 2 through 5	Once daily	5 days
	Adult: 500 mg on day 1; 250 mg on days 2 through 5	Once daily	5 days
Amoxicillin-clavulanate potassium (Augmentin)	Child: 40 mg per kg per day	Two or three divided doses	10 days
	Adult: 500 to 875 mg	Two times daily	10 days
Cefadroxil (Duricef)	Child: 30 mg per kg per day	Two divided doses	10 days
	Adult: 1 g	Once daily	10 days
Cephalexin (Keflex)	Child: 25 to 50 mg per kg per day	Two to four divided doses	10 days
	Adult: 500 mg	Two times daily	10 days

A. Penicillin is the drug of choice for streptococcal pharyngitis. This antibiotic has efficacy and safety, a narrow spectrum of activity and low cost. About 10 percent of patients are allergic to penicillin. Cure rates similar for 250 mg of penicillin V given two, three or four times daily. The use of intramuscularly administered penicillin may overcome compliance problems.

B. Alternatives to Penicillin

1. Amoxicillin

    a. In children, the cure rates for amoxicillin given once daily for 10 days are similar to those for penicillin V. The absorption of amoxicillin is unaffected by the ingestion of food.

    b. Amoxicillin is less expensive and has a narrower spectrum of antimicrobial activity than the once-daily antibiotics. Suspensions of this drug taste better than penicillin V suspensions, and chewable tablets are available. However, gastrointestinal side effects and skin rash may be more common with amoxicillin.

2. Macrolides

    a. Erythromycin is recommended in patients with penicillin allergy. Because erythromycin estolate is hepatotoxic in adults, erythromycin ethylsuccinate may be used. Erythromycin is absorbed better when it is given with food. About 15 to 20 percent of patients cannot tolerate the gastrointestinal side effects of erythromycin.

    b. Azithromycin (Zithromax) allows once-daily dosing and a shorter treatment course of five-days. Azithromycin is associated with a low incidence of gastrointestinal side effects.

3. Cephalosporins

    a. A 10-day course of a cephalosporin has been shown to be superior to penicillin. The overall bacteriologic cure rate for cephalosporins is 92 percent, compared with 84 percent for penicillin.

    b. Cephalosporins have a broader spectrum of activity than penicillin V. Unlike penicillin, cephalosporins are resistant to degradation from beta-lactamase. First-generation agents such as cefadroxil (Duricef) and cephalexin (Keflex, Keftab) are preferable to second- or third-generation agents.

    c. Cephalosporins are reserved for patients with relapse or recurrence of streptococcal pharyngitis.

   4. Amoxicillin-clavulanate (Augmentin) is resistant to degradation from beta-lactamase produced by copathogens. Amoxicillin-clavulanate is often used to treat recurrent streptococcal pharyngitis. Its major adverse effect is diarrhea.

V. Management Issues
  A. Treatment Failure and Reinfection. Patients who do not comply with a 10-day course of penicillin should be offered intramuscular penicillin or a once-daily oral macrolide or cephalosporin. Patients with clinical failure should be treated with amoxicillin-clavulanate, a cephalosporin, or a macrolide.
  B. Contagion. Patients with streptococcal pharyngitis are considered contagious until they have been taking an antibiotic for 24 hours. Children should not go back to day-care or school until their temperature returns to normal and they have had at least 24 hours of antibiotic therapy.

References, see page 164.

Acute Conjunctivitis

Conjunctivitis is defined as inflammation of the conjunctiva; it is usually caused by infection or allergy. It is often referred to as "pink eye."

I. Etiology
  A. Neonatal conjunctivitis occurs in 1.6-12% of newborns. The most common cause is chemical irritation from antimicrobial prophylaxis against bacterial infection, followed by Chlamydia trachomatis infection. Haemophilus influenzae and Streptococcus pneumoniae may also cause infection in newborns.
  B. Rarely, gram-negative organisms such as Escherichia coli, Klebsiella, or Pseudomonas sp can cause neonatal conjunctivitis. Neisseria gonorrhoeae is an unusual cause of neonatal conjunctivitis because of the use of ocular prophylaxis.
  C. Herpes simplex can cause neonatal keratoconjunctivitis; however, it is almost always associated with infection of the skin and mucous membranes, or with disseminated disease.
  D. In older infants and children, H influenzae is by far the most common identifiable cause of conjunctivitis, causing 40-50% of episodes. S pneumoniae accounts for 10% of cases, and Moraxella catarrhalis is the third most common cause.
  E. Adenovirus is the most important viral cause of acute conjunctivitis. This organism often causes epidemics of acute conjunctivitis. It causes 20% of childhood conjunctivitis (most occurring in the fall and winter months).

II. Clinical presentation
  A. In the first day of life, conjunctivitis is usually caused by chemical conjunctivitis secondary to ocular prophylaxis.
  B. Three to 5 days after birth, gonococcal conjunctivitis is the most common cause of conjunctivitis.
  C. After the first week of life and throughout the first month, chlamydia is the most frequent cause of conjunctivitis. Severe cases are associated with a thick mucopurulent discharge and pseudomembrane formation.
  D. Gonococcal conjunctivitis can present as typical bacterial conjunctivitis, or as a hyperacute conjunctivitis with profuse purulent discharge. There often is severe edema of both lids.
  E. In the older infant and child, both viral and bacterial conjunctivitis may present with an acutely inflamed eye. Typically, there is conjunctival erythema, with occasional lid edema. Exudate often accumulates during the night.

    F. Many patients who have both adenoviral conjunctivitis and pharyngitis also are febrile. The triad of pharyngitis, conjunctivitis, and fever has been termed pharyngoconjunctival fever.

III. Diagnosis

  A. Neonates

    1. In cases of neonatal conjunctivitis, a Gram stain and culture should be obtained to exclude N gonorrhoeae conjunctivitis.

    2. Chlamydia trachomatis antigen detection assays have a sensitivity and specificity of 90%.

  B. Infants and older children. Outside the neonatal period, a Gram stain is usually not needed unless the conjunctivitis lasts longer than 7 days. The presence of vesicles or superficial corneal ulcerations suggests herpetic keratoconjunctivitis.

IV. Differential diagnosis of conjunctivitis

  A. Systemic diseases. Most cases of red eye in children are caused by acute conjunctivitis, allergy, or trauma; however, Kawasaki disease, Lyme disease, leptospirosis, juvenile rheumatoid arthritis, and Stevens-Johnson syndrome may cause conjunctivitis. Glaucoma is a significant cause of a red eye in adults; however, it is rare in children.

  B. Allergic conjunctivitis

    1. Allergic eye disease is characterized by pronounced ocular itching, redness, tearing, and photophobia. This recurrent disease has seasonal exacerbations in the spring, summer, and fall. Children who have allergic conjunctivitis often have other atopic diseases (rhinitis, eczema, asthma) and a positive family history.

    2. Treatment

      a. Topical decongestants: Naphazoline 0.1% (Naphcon), phenylephrine (Neo-Synephrine), and oxymetazoline (OcuClear, Visine LR) may be used qid, alone or in combination with ophthalmic antihistamines, such as antazoline (Vasocon-A) or pheniramine maleate (Naph-Con-A).

      b. Topical Iodoxamide (Alomide) 0.1% ophthalmic solution, 1-2 drops qid, is helpful in more severe cases.

      c. Topical corticosteroids are helpful, but long-term use is not recommended; dexamethasone (Decadron) 1-2 drops tid-qid.

V. Treatment of acute infectious conjunctivitis

  A. Gonococcal ophthalmia neonatorum is treated with ceftriaxone (50 mg/kg/day IV/IM q24h) or cefotaxime (100 mg/kg/day IV/IM q12h) for 7 days.

  B. Neonatal conjunctivitis caused by C trachomatis is treated with erythromycin 50 mg/kg/day PO divided in 4 doses for 14 days.

  C. Bacterial conjunctivitis among older infants and children is treated with polymyxin-bacitracin (Polysporin) ointment, applied to affected eye tid.

References, see page 164.

Cat and Dog Bites

Bite wounds account for approximately 1% of all emergency department visits: 10% of victims require suturing and 1-2% require hospitalization.

I. Pathophysiology

  A. Dog bites account for 80-90% of animal bites. Infection develops in 15-20% of dog bite wounds.

  B. Cat bites account for 15% of animal bites. Cat bites usually present as puncture wounds, of which 30-40% become infected.

II. **Clinical evaluation of bite wounds**
   A. **The circumstances of the injury** should be documented, and the animal's immunization status should be determined. Determine whether the animal was provoked and to record the time of the injury.
   B. The patient's tetanus immunization status, current medications and allergies, history of chronic illness, or immunocompromising conditions should be assessed. The wound is measured and classified as a laceration, puncture, crush injury or avulsion. Wounds are evaluated for injuries to tendons, joint spaces, blood vessels, nerves, or bone. A neurovascular examination and an assessment of wound depth should be completed.
   C. **Photographs** of the wound should be obtained if disfigurement has occurred or if litigation is anticipated.
III. **Laboratory and radiologic evaluation**
   A. **Radiographs** should be taken if there is considerable edema and tenderness around the wound or if bony penetration or foreign bodies are suspected.
   B. **Wounds seen within 8 to 24 hours after injury**, that have no signs of infection, do not require culture. If infection is present, aerobic and anaerobic cultures should be obtained.
IV. **Microbiology**
   A. **Bite wounds** usually have a polymicrobial contamination.
   B. **Pasteurella Multocida** is a gram-negative aerobe present in the oropharynx of dogs and cats. It is found in 20-30% of dog bite wounds and more than 50% of cat bite wounds.

Microorganisms Isolated from Infected Dog and Cat Bite Wounds	
Aerobes. Afipia felis, Capnocytophaga canimorsus, Eikenella corrodens, Enterobacter species, Flavobacterium species, Haemophilus aphrophilus, Moraxella species, Neisseria species, Pasteurella multocida, Pseudomonas species, Staphylococcus aureus, Staphylococcus epidermidis, Staphylococcus intermedius, Streptococci: alpha-hemolytic, beta-hemolytic, gamma-hemolytic	**Anaerobes.** Actinomyces, Bacteroides species, Eubacterium species, Fusobacterium species, Leptotrichia buccalis, Veillonella parvula
	Unusual Pathogens. Blastomyces dermatitidis, Francisella tularensis

V. **Management of dog and cat bites**
   A. **Wound care**
      1. The wound should be cleansed with 1% povidone iodine solution (Betadine), and irrigated with normal saline with a 20- to 50-mL syringe with an Angiocath. Devitalized, crushed tissue should be sharply débrided.
      2. Deep puncture wounds, wounds examined more than 24 hours after injury, clinically infected wounds, and bites of the hand should not be closed primarily.
      3. Low-risk wounds seen within 24 hours after injury may be sutured; uninfected high-risk wounds seen 72 hours after initial injury may undergo delayed primary closure. Bites to the face and head have a good outcome and may be closed primarily.
   B. **Antimicrobial therapy**
      1. Prophylactic antibiotics are recommended for wounds that have a high risk of infection. Prophylactic antibiotic treatment is given for 3-7 days.
      2. **High-risk bite wounds requiring prophylactic antibiotics**
         a. Full-thickness puncture wounds, severe crush injury and/or edema, wounds requiring debridement.

    b. Cat bite wounds.
    c. Bite wounds to the hand, foot or face; bone, joint, tendon or ligament, or wound adjacent to a prosthetic joint.
    d. Underlying diabetes, liver or pulmonary disease, history of splenectomy, malignancy, acquired immunodeficiency syndrome, or other immunocompromising condition.

Prophylactic Antibiotics for Dog and Cat Bites	
Outpatient Antibiotics	
Cephalexin (Keflex)	**Adults:** 500 mg qid **Children:** 40 mg/kg/d PO qid
Doxycycline (Vibramycin)	**Adults:** 100 mg bid **Children:** 2-4 mg/kg/day, in divided doses bid
Amoxicillin/clavulanate (Augmentin)	**Adults:** 500 mg tid **Children:** 40 mg amoxicillin/kg/day, in divided doses tid
Ceftriaxone (Rocephin)	**Adults:** 1 g every 24 hours IM or IV **Children:** 50 mg/kg/d qd
Penicillin V	**Adults:** 500 mg qid **Children:** 50 mg/kg/day, in divided doses q6-8h
Amoxicillin	**Adults:** 500 mg tid **Children:** 40 mg/kg/d, in divided doses tid
Intravenous Antibiotic of choice	
Cefoxitin (Mefoxin)	**Adults:** 1-2 g q4-8h **Children:** 25-50 mg/kg/day, in divided doses q6h
Alternative Intravenous Antibiotics	
Ampicillin/sulbactam (Unasyn)	**Adults:** 1.5-3.0 g q6h
Ticarcillin-clavulanate (Timentin)	**Adults:** 3.1 g q6h
Ceftriaxone (Rocephin)	**Adults:** 1-2 g q24h **Children:** 50-100 mg/kg/day, in divided doses q24h

  C. Treatment of infected wounds. Infected bite wounds are treated with amoxicillin/clavulanate (Augmentin). Cellulitis is treated for 10-14 days.
  D. Rabies immunoprophylaxis
    1. The incidence of rabies in persons who have been bitten by a dog is very low because most dogs have been vaccinated. An untreated person has a less than 20% chance of contracting rabies from the bite of a rabid animal. However, if rabies is contracted, the mortality rate is 100%.
    2. Wild animals (raccoons, skunks, bats) are the most common source of rabies. Rabies is transmitted when the saliva of an infected animal comes into contact

with the broken skin or mucosa of another mammal. The incubation period ranges from 10 days to one year.

   3. If rabies infection is suspected, rabies prophylaxis is administered as follows:
      a. **Rabies immune globulin (RIG),** 20 IU/kg, IM (separate from human diploid cell vaccine below).
      b. **Human diploid cell vaccine (HDCV),** 1 cc IM (not gluteal) given on days 1, 3, 7, 14, and 28.

   E. **Tetanus Immunization.** Animal bites should be regarded as tetanus prone, although tetanus infection resulting from cat and dog bites is rare.

References, see page 164.

Cervical Adenopathy

Cervical lymph gland enlargement commonly occurs in children. In most cases the enlargement is a transient response to a benign local or generalized viral infection. Almost all children have small palpable cervical, axillary, and inguinal nodes. About 5% have small palpable suboccipital nodes. Distinctly uncommon are palpable postauricular, supraclavicular, epitrochlear, or popliteal nodes.

I. **Pathophysiology**
   A. Often the cause of the adenopathy is obvious, such as with lymph glands draining an obvious source of infection. Malignancy is suggested by painless adenopathy in the posterior or lower cervical chains, particularly in older children.
   B. Almost all adenopathy in the anterior cervical triangle (anterior to the sternomastoid muscle) is benign. Fifty percent of masses in the posterior triangle are malignant.

II. **Etiology and epidemiology**
   A. **Infection** is the most common cause of cervical adenopathy in children.
   B. **Viral agents** are the most common infectious agents causing cervical adenopathy. Human herpesvirus 6, adenoviruses, herpes simplex virus, rubella, mumps virus, Epstein-Barr, cytomegalovirus, varicella, human immunodeficiency virus and respiratory viruses may cause cervical adenitis.
   C. **Bacterial infection** may be caused by oropharyngeal flora (anaerobes, group B streptococci, Staphylococcus aureus, Streptococcus pyogenes [GABS], atypical mycobacteria, Haemophilus sp, Actinomyces israelii, or Nocardia sp).
   D. **Staphylococcus aureus and group A beta-hemolytic streptococci** account for 65-89% of acute unilateral infectious cervical adenitis in children. The majority occur in children ages 1 to 4 years.
   E. **Group A beta-hemolytic Streptococci, Mycobacterium tuberculosis, or corynebacterium diphtheriae** may result form person-to-person spread by airborne droplets.
   F. **Contact with domestic or wild animals or with feeding insects** may result in lymphadenitis due to Toxoplasma gondii, Francisella tularensis, Yersinia pestis, Rochalimaea henselae, or Pasteurella multocida.
   G. **Cat-scratch disease (Bartonella henselae)** most often occurs after a lick or scratch from a cat or dog, or inoculation by a wood splinter, pin, fish hook, cactus spike, or porcupine quill.

Infectious Etiologies of Cervical Adenitis			
Bacterial	**Viral**	**Fungal/protozoal**	**Other**
Localized Acute			
Staphylococcus aureus *Streptococcus pyogenes* Group B streptococcus Anaerobes *Francisella tularensis*	Rubella Adenoviruses Herpes simplex virus Mumps Human herpes- virus 6	Toxoplasmosis Histoplasmosis	Kawasaki syndrome Rickettsial pox
Subacute or Chronic			
Tuberculosis Atypical mycobacteria Cat-scratch disease	Syphilis Actinomycosis Nocardiosis		Brucellosis
Generalized			
Syphilis Tuberculosis Scarlet fever Typhoid fever Leptospirosis Brucellosis virus	HIV Epstein-Barr Cytomegalovirus Measles Rubella Varicella Adenovirus	Histoplasmosis Toxoplasmosis	Rickettsial Scrub typhus

H. **Toxoplasma gondii** may result from contact with cat feces, undercooked meat, or contaminated vegetables.

I. **Francisella tularensis** may be transmitted by direct contact with infected animals or their carcasses, by ingestion of water contaminated by animals, or by bites of ticks, deer flies, mosquitoes, or mites.

J. **Brucellosis** may result from contact with or ingestion of contaminated meat or dairy products, which can include those from cattle, swine, goats, dogs, or sheep.

K. **Leptospirosis** results most often from contact with water or soil contaminated by cats, dogs, rodents, or livestock.

L. **Pasteurella multocida** is an aerobic coccobacillus found in the normal flora of the mouth of many animals and occasionally of humans.

M. **Atypical mycobacterial infections** occur typically in rural Caucasian children, 1 to 4 years of age, who have no history of exposure to tuberculosis. Involvement usually is unilateral and associated with a normal chest radiograph and a normal purified protein derivative (PPD) skin test.

N. **Mycobacterium tuberculosis** generally causes tubercular cervical adenitis in children who are urban and black, have a history of exposure to tuberculosis, have an abnormal chest radiograph, unilateral or bilateral involvement, and an abnormal PPD.

O. **Kawasaki syndrome** may cause unilateral cervical lymphadenopathy in infants and toddlers.

Organism Associated with Infectious Cervical Lymphadenitis
Neonates
Staphylococcus aureus Group B streptococcal "cellulitis-adenitis" syndrome
Infancy
As above Kawasaki syndrome
1 to 4 Years
Staphylococcus aureus Streptococcus pyogenes Atypical mycobacteria
5 to 15 years
Anaerobic bacteria Toxoplasmosis Cat-scratch disease Tuberculosis

II. **Clinical evaluation of cervical adenopathy**
   A. **Seventy to 80% of acute unilateral cervical adenitis cases**, caused by GABS or staphylococcal infection, occur in those aged 1 to 4 years who frequently have a history of upper respiratory symptoms. The submandibular nodes are involved most commonly.
   B. **Group A beta-hemolytic streptococcal** disease should be suspected when impetigo or pharyngitis is present.
   C. **Staphylococcus aureus and group B streptococci** are the most common causes of cervical lymphadenitis in newborn infants. In older infants whose mean age is 5 weeks, group B streptococcus causes the "cellulitis-adenitis" syndrome.
   D. **A papular or pustular lesion** distal to the adenopathy, suggesting an inoculation site, should lead to consideration of tularemia, Nocardia, actinomycosis, plague, cutaneous diphtheria, and cat-scratch disease.
   E. **Tularemia** is a disease of acute onset associated with fever, chills, and headaches. It is characterized by tender swollen lymph nodes and a painful swollen papule, which develops distal to the involved nodes. The papule then ruptures to form an ulcer. Fifty percent of the lymph nodes will suppurate and drain while the other 50% remain enlarged and tender for several months.
   F. **Toxoplasmosis** most often is an asymptomatic infection accounting for 3-7% of significant adenopathy. The lymph nodes are discrete, rarely more than 3 cm in diameter, usually not tender, and do not suppurate. The clinical course is self-limited, lasting for up to 12 months.
   G. **Cat-scratch disease** presents as a small papule that appears at the inoculation site 7 to 12 days after inoculation. Over the next 4 weeks, regional lymphadenitis appears. The involved regional lymph nodes are tender, warm, red, and indurated; up to 40% may suppurate. The lymphadenitis runs an indolent course of 4 to 6 weeks.
   H. **Yersinia pestis** causes acute onset of fever, chills, headache, and weakness, which may be accompanied by a papule at the inoculation site. In bubonic plague,

large, fixed, edematous and exquisitely tender nodes develop at one site.

I. **Brucellosis**, causes mild cervical or inguinal adenopathy, malaise, and fever within 1 week to several months of ingesting or inhaling the organism.

J. **Pasteurella multocida** infections cause an acute edematous cellulitis of the inoculation site, with fever, headache, and regional adenopathy.

IV. Diagnosis of cervical adenopathy

A. **Acute pyogenic bacterial infection** most often will be associated with an acute onset of 5 days or less, tender, enlarged nodes, and fever. The adenopathy may be bilateral if pharyngitis was the primary focus or unilateral if the focus is a dental or skin abscess. Associated generalized adenopathy suggests a generalized infection.

B. **Subacute or chronic adenopathy.** When the involved nodes are well localized, nontender, and unilateral, a granulomatous infection or malignancy is most likely.

    1. A history of exposure to an individual who has tuberculosis or to ticks or other insects, cats, rodents, or other wild animals may suggest an etiology. If the adenopathy is generalized, tuberculosis, brucellosis, and histoplasmosis are more likely.

    2. If the adenopathy is unilateral, an atypical mycobacterial infection or cat-scratch disease is more likely.

C. **Physical examination.** Characteristics of the involved nodes and possible foci of infection or inoculate should be assessed. Fever, generalized adenopathy, hepatosplenomegaly, rash, joint swelling, and pulmonary findings should be sought.

D. **Tumors**, particularly neuroblastomas in younger children and lymphomas in older children, should be considered when evaluating any subacute or chronic painless, firm, and noninflamed cervical mass. A malignancy is of particular concern in older children when the node is in the posterior triangle or extends across the sternomastoid muscle to involve the anterior triangle.

V. Aspiration, biopsy, and laboratory tests

A. **A specific diagnosis** of cervical adenitis depends either on demonstration of the organism by Gram stain, culture of aspirated or biopsied tissue, elevated IgM antibody titers, or skin testing. A complete blood count, erythrocyte sedimentation rate, liver function tests, or radiographic studies may help define the extent of involvement.

B. **Needle aspiration** of acutely inflamed nodes should be performed if 48 hours of antimicrobial therapy has failed, or if the infection is severe enough to require parenteral therapy.

C. **Aspiration.** After cleansing and anesthetizing the skin, the aspiration is performed with a 18- to 20-gauge needle and a 10- to 20-cc syringe. If no material is aspirated 1 to 2 mL of sterile saline is injected and reaspirated.

D. **Nodes should be incised and drained** if pus is demonstrated on needle aspiration.

E. **Excisional node biopsy** should be performed for adenopathy suggestive of a malignancy. Excisional biopsy or incision and drainage are indicated for noninflamed hard nodes, nodes fixed to adjacent structures (particularly in the posterior triangle) and in older children, who have an increased incidence of lymphoma.

VI. Management of acute pyogenic bacterial lymphadenitis

Treatment of Acute Pyogenic Bacterial Lymphadenitis
Symptomatic Therapy
1. Apply warm, moist dressings 2. Prescribe analgesics 3. Incise and drain nodes that have suppuration
Antimicrobial Therapy

Suspected staphylococcal/group A and B streptococcal disease
  Cellulitis or marked enlargement, moderate-to-severe systemic symptoms, or in
    infants 1 mo of age:
    IV Nafcillin (Nafcil) 150 mg/kg day or
    IV Cefazolin (Ancef) 150 mg/kg/day after aspiration of node
  Suppuration:
    IV antibiotics as above and incision and drainage
  No prominent systemic symptoms, cellulitis, or suppuration:
    Dicloxacillin (Dynapen) 25 mg/kg/day or
    Cephalexin (Keflex) 50 mg/kg/day or
    Clindamycin (Cleocin) 30 mg/kg/day
Suspected anaerobic infection with dental or periodontal disease, include:
  Penicillin V 50 mg/kg/day or
  Clindamycin (Cleocin) 30 mg/kg/day or
Group A streptococcal infection
  Aqueous penicillin G 50 000 IU/kg/day IV or
  Penicillin V 50 mg/kg/day PO or
  Cephalexin 50 mg/kg/day PO or erythromycin ethylsuccinate 40 mg/kg/day PO
Group B streptococcal disease in infants
  Aqueous penicillin G 200 000 IU/kg/day IV, if sensitive.

References, see page 164.

Intestinal Helminths

Intestinal helminth infestations most commonly affect travelers, migrant laborers, refugees, children of foreign adoptions, and the homeless. These parasitic infections are associated with day care centers and overseas travel.

I. Clinical evaluation
   A. **Intestinal helminth infections are usually asymptomatic**, but serious infections may cause symptoms ranging from abdominal discomfort to severe pain. Anorexia, nausea, diarrhea, pruritus, rectal prolapse, bowel obstruction, and death may occur. Hives and eosinophilia may develop, and the worms may sometimes spontaneously exit the body through the anus.
   B. **Stool examination.** Examination of the stool for ova and parasites is the most important test for helminthic infection. Stools are collected using plastic wrap under the toilet seat. Fresh stool may also be obtained by rectal examination.

II. Enterobiasis
   A. **The pinworm (Enterobius vermicularis)** is the most common helminth. Pinworms present as anal pruritus in irritable children. The disorder tends to occur in temperate climates. Many patients are asymptomatic. Heavier infections may cause insomnia,

restlessness, vulvovaginitis, loss of appetite, and intractable anal itching.
- **B.** Pinworms are about 10 mm in length. The female worm has a pin-shaped tail. At night, worms migrate through the anus, then deposit their eggs and die on the perianal skin. Microscopic eggs infest clothing, bedding, and other surfaces, often spreading to the entire family.
- **C.** Pinworms are diagnosed by examining the perianal skin. The stool is usually negative for ova and worms. To obtain the eggs, a tongue blade covered with clear tape is placed sticky-side down over the perianal skin in the morning. Specimens are collected on three separate mornings, then taped to glass slides and taken to a laboratory for examination.
- **D.** The elongate, colorless eggs measure 50 to 60 μm and are flattened on one side. Worms may also be visualized if the anus is examined late at night or early in the morning.
- **E. Treatment**
  1. **Mebendazole (Vermox)**, one 100-mg tablet orally, is safe and effective. A second dose is given 10 days later. The entire family is treated.
  2. Infested clothing and bedding are washed and fingernails should be kept trimmed, and the perianal area kept clean. Dogs and cats do not spread this infection. Relapses are common.

III. Ascariasis
- **A. Roundworms (Ascaris lumbricoides)** measure up to 18 inches in length. The infection is fairly common in the rural southeastern United States and is frequent among immigrants. A. lumbricoides only infests humans.
- **B.** Ascaris eggs reach the soil in feces, and they may persist in the soil for more than a decade until they are accidentally consumed. In the gut, worms may cause intestinal obstruction. However, most patients experience only vague abdominal discomfort or nausea.
- **C. Treatment**
  1. **Mebendazole (Vermox)**, 100 mg bid for three days.
  2. A follow-up examination of stool for ova and parasites should be performed in two months. Family screening is recommended.

IV. Trichuriasis
- **A. Whipworm (Trichuris trichiura)** infestation is less common than Ascaris infestation, occurring in the southeastern states and in foreign immigrants.
- **B.** Whipworm eggs incubate in the soil. When swallowed, they travel to the colon.
- **C.** Adult whipworms are 30-50 μm in length, with a thread-like anterior portion. They can live in the intestine and produce eggs for several years, causing mild blood loss and symptoms similar to proctitis and inflammatory bowel disease. Rectal prolapse, diarrhea, loss of appetite, and hives may occur.
- **D.** Treatment of trichuriasis is the same as for ascariasis.

V. Less common parasites
- **A. Hookworms**
  1. Hookworms develop in the soil from eggs in feces. The larvae are capable of penetrating the bare feet and causing a pruritic rash. The larvae eventually reach the small intestine.
  2. Adult hookworms are about 10 μm in length, with a hooked anterior end, which they use to consume 0.03-0.15 mL of blood per day for 10 to 15 years. Manifestations include iron deficiency anemia, chronic fatigue, geophagia, failure to thrive, and depression.
  3. Treatment consists of mebendazole as described above and iron supplementation.
- **B. Strongyloidiasis**
  1. Filariform larvae are capable of penetrating intact skin, persisting for 40 years or more in the small intestine. It can also be spread in feces or as a sexually

transmitted disease. Persistent unexplained eosinophilia in a patient from a region where Strongyloides infection is endemic should prompt serologic testing because stool specimens are often negative.

   2. Symptoms are usually absent but may include pruritus, pneumonia, abdominal cramping, and colitis. Treatment consists of thiabendazole (Mintezol).

C. Tapeworms
   1. **Beef tapeworm** is transmitted by inadequately cooked beef, reaching up to 10 to 15 feet in length in the gut. Diagnosis is made by passage of ribbon-like tapeworm segments or by finding the eggs in a stool.
   2. **Pork tapeworm** is far more dangerous than T. saginata since its eggs can cause cysticercosis, the invasion of human tissue by larval forms. In severe cases, the larvae may invade the central nervous system, causing neurocysticercosis.
      a. Pork tapeworm is found in immigrants from Central and South America. Patients with neurocysticercosis frequently present with seizures.
      b. This diagnosis should be considered in the evaluation of a patient from Central or South America with a new-onset seizure disorder.
   3. **Dwarf tapeworm** is the most common tapeworm in the U.S. This tapeworm is 1 inch in length. Ingestion of food contaminated with mouse droppings may spread the infection. H. nana infection may cycle in immigrant children for years.
   4. **Fish tapeworm** is occasionally transmitted by undercooked fish, especially from the Great Lakes region. It can occasionally causes megaloblastic anemia.
   5. **Treatment of all tapeworms** consists of praziquantel (Biltricide) or niclosamide (Niclocide).

References, see page 164.

Orbital and Periorbital Cellulitis

Periorbital cellulitis is a bacterial infection of the skin and structures superficial to the orbit; orbital cellulitis is a bacterial infection of the orbit.

I. Pathogenesis of periorbital cellulitis
   A. The most common causes of eyelid redness and swelling are allergy, trauma, and insect stings or bites. Periorbital cellulitis usually occurs after the skin near the eye has been broken by trauma, an insect bite, or infection with herpes simplex or varicella zoster viruses. The organisms that most frequently cause periorbital cellulitis following trauma are Staphylococcus aureus and Streptococcus pyogenes (group A beta-hemolytic streptococci).
   B. A bacterial pathogen is identified in only 30% of cases of periorbital cellulitis, and the pathogen is isolated from the blood in about two thirds of these cases.
   C. Since the introduction of H influenzae type b conjugate vaccines (HbCV), Hib disease accounts for fewer than 15% of periorbital cellulitis. A child who has received a second dose of HbCV more than 1 week before the onset of eyelid swelling is very unlikely to have HIB disease.
II. Pathogenesis of orbital cellulitis
   A. Orbital cellulitis may progress to subperiosteal abscess, orbital abscess, and cavernous sinus thrombosis.
   B. About one-fourth of isolates are S aureus; one-fifth, S pyogenes; one-fifth, HiB; one-tenth, S pneumoniae; one-tenth, anaerobic bacteria; and the remaining 15%, other bacteria.
III. Clinical evaluation
   A. Periorbital cellulitis usually occurs in children younger than 2 years of age. Clinical findings include a temperature of 39°C or more and a peripheral white blood cell

count of greater than 15,000/mm³.

B. Periorbital and orbital cellulitis cause eyelid swelling, with the swelling being unilateral in 95-98% of cases. Virtually all involved eyelids will be erythematous or violaceous.

C. Signs of trauma or local infection are observed in one-third of patients. When conjunctival inflammation, a purulent discharge, and bilateral lid involvement are present, the cause is much more likely to be conjunctivitis, rather than periorbital or orbital cellulitis.

D. **Globe displacement (proptosis), abnormal movement (ophthalmoplegia), or pain on movement** should be sought, and visual acuity should be tested.

E. **Laboratory evaluation**

   1. **White blood cell count** greater than 15,000/mm³ suggests bacteremic disease.

   2. **Lumbar puncture** should be performed on all children younger than 1 year of age who have not had at least two doses of H influenzae B vaccine.

   3. **Blood culture for bacterial pathogens** should be obtained.

IV. **Treatment**

   A. **Orbital cellulitis.** Children who have signs of orbital cellulitis should be hospitalized, and antimicrobial therapy should consist of a third-generation cephalosporin, such as ceftriaxone (50 mg/kg qd IM or IV) or cefotaxime (50 mg/kg/dose q6h IV), plus clindamycin (10 mg/kg/dose q8h IV).

   B. **Periorbital cellulitis**

      1. Periorbital cellulitis can be managed on an outpatient basis if there is no orbital involvement and the child does not appear toxic.

      2. Ceftriaxone (50 mg/kg, not to exceed 1 g) is given IM or IV. If the blood culture remains negative, the child may be started on a broad-spectrum oral agent such as ampicillin/clavulanate (Augmentin) or trimethoprim/sulfamethoxazole (Bactrim) to complete a 7- to 10-day course of therapy.

References, see page 164.

Tuberculosis

The number of cases of tuberculosis in children younger than five years of age in cities has increased 94.3% in the last four years.

I. **Natural history of tuberculosis**

   A. Tuberculosis infection is initiated by the inhalation of organisms into the lung. During an incubation period, that lasts 2 to 10 weeks, the organisms spread to the hilar lymph nodes. This condition is considered primary tuberculosis. During the incubation period, the purified protein derivative (PPD) test usually becomes positive.

   B. **Primary tuberculosis** is often completely asymptomatic, and the chest radiograph may be only minimally abnormal, with hilar adenopathy, and/or small parenchymal infiltrates. Healed primary tuberculosis may leave calcified deposits in the lung parenchyma and/or hilum.

   C. **Extrapulmonary disease** is more common in children than in adults. In children, 25% of tuberculosis disease is extrapulmonary. Children and young adolescents are more likely than adults to have tuberculous meningitis, miliary tuberculosis, adenitis, and bone and joint infections.

   D. **Reactivation.** Children who do not have clinical disease, but who harbor a reservoir of quiescent organisms may develop tuberculous disease later in life. Reactivation is most likely to occur during adolescence, during an episode of immunosuppression, in the presence of chronic disease, or in the elderly.

II. Diagnosis of tuberculosis in children

A. Children exposed to tuberculosis

1. All household contacts of adults with active disease should be tested by PPD. Thirty to 50% of all household contacts of infectious adults will have a positive PPD.

2. Children who are known contacts and who are PPD negative, should receive prophylactic therapy, usually isoniazid (Laniazid), 10 mg/kg/day. The PPD is repeated in 3 months to check for conversion to a positive PPD test, which would indicate infection. If the repeat PPD test remains negative, the child is assumed not to be infected, and prophylactic therapy can be discontinued. If the repeat PPD test is positive, the child should be treated for 9 months.

3. Any child with a positive PPD test should be evaluated for active pulmonary and extrapulmonary tuberculosis with a history and physical examination and posteroanterior and lateral chest radiographs. The source of the child's infection should be determined. The susceptibility of the source case's M. tuberculosis strain is considered in selecting a prophylactic or treatment regimen. Contact with the person with contagious tuberculosis who infected the child must be prevented until the source case is no longer infectious.

B. Children at risk for infection

1. A PPD test is recommended for children in high-risk groups. A screening PPD test of 5 tuberculin units can be placed before a dose of measles-mumps-rubella (MMR) vaccine, simultaneously with the MMR vaccine dose, or 6 weeks after the MMR vaccine dose. A false-negative PPD test may occur within 6 weeks of an MMR vaccination, because of transient immunosuppression from the live MMR vaccine.

2. The size of the PPD reaction determined to be positive varies with the risk of tuberculous infection. The diameter of the induration is measured 48 to 72 hours after PPD placement. A positive PPD test requires an evaluation for tuberculous disease.

Criteria for a Positive PPD Test in Children

Reaction of 5 mm or more
Children suspected of having tuberculosis (chest x-ray consistent with active or previously active tuberculosis; clinical signs of tuberculosis)
Children in close contact with persons who have known or suspected infectious tuberculosis
Children with immunosuppressive conditions (HIV infection, corticosteroid therapy)

Reaction of 10 mm or more
Children younger than 4 years of age
Children born in, or whose parents were born in, regions where tuberculosis is highly prevalent
Children frequently exposed to adults who are HIV infected, homeless persons, IV and other street drug users, poor and medically indigent city dwellers, residents of nursing homes, incarcerated or institutionalized persons, and migrant farm workers
Children with other medical risk factors (Hodgkin's disease, lymphoma, diabetes mellitus, chronic renal failure)

Reaction of 15 mm or more
Children older than 4 years without any risk factors

---

3. Previous vaccination with bacille Calmette-Guerin (BCG) vaccine does not change the interpretation of the PPD test.

4. High tuberculous infection rates occur in Southeast Asia, Africa, Eastern

Mediterranean countries, Western Pacific countries, Mexico, the Caribbean, and South and Central America.

C. **Clinical evidence suggestive of tuberculosis**. Tuberculosis must be considered when a child presents with pneumonia that is unresponsive to antibiotic treatment, "aseptic" meningitis, joint or bone infection, hilar or cervical adenopathy, or pleural effusion.

III. **Evaluation of tuberculosis in children**

A. The work-up for a child with a positive PPD test or suspected tuberculosis includes the following:

1. **History.** Risk factors for exposure to tuberculosis; symptoms of tuberculosis; adult source case.

2. **Physical examination.** Adenopathy, positive respiratory system findings, bone or joint disease, meningitis.

3. **Diagnostic tests**

a. Chest x-ray (posteroanterior and lateral).

b. Gastric aspirates in children who are too young to produce a deep sputum sample

c. Sputum collection or induction in children who are able to produce a deep sputum sample.

d. Cultures and smears of appropriate body fluids in children with suspected extrapulmonary tuberculosis.

IV. **Treatment of active tuberculosis**

A. Treatments should be directly observed to ensure compliance. If possible, the susceptibility results of the adult source case should guide the medication choice. If the organism may be resistant to one of the standard medications, ethambutol (Myambutol) (or streptomycin in children too young for visual acuity testing) should be included.

B. Drug-resistant tuberculosis should be suspected in children who are exposed to immigrants from Asia, Africa and Latin America, children who live in large cities, or who are from areas in which isoniazid resistance occurs in more than 4% of cases, children who are homeless, children who have previously been treated for tuberculosis, and children who are exposed to adults at high risk for tuberculosis.

Treatment Regimens for Active Tuberculosis		
Type of Disease	**Primary Regimen**	**Comments**
Pulmonary disease	Two months of isoniazid, 10-15 mg/kg/day, max 300 mg/day; rifampin (Rifadin), 10-20 mg/kg/day, max 600 mg/day; and pyrazinamide, 20-40 mg/kg/day, max 2.0 g/day, followed by 4 months of daily or twice-weekly isoniazid and rifampin	Medications can be given 2 or 3 times/week under direct observation in the initial phase
Extrapulmonary disease, except meningitis, miliary disease and bone/joint disease	Same as for pulmonary disease	

Type of Disease	Primary Regimen	Comments
Meningitis, miliary disease, and bone/joint disease	Two months of daily isoniazid, rifampin, pyrazinamide and streptomycin, followed by 10 months of daily or twice-weekly isoniazid and rifampin	

Treatment of latent tuberculosis infection
A. Children with a positive PPD test, but no signs of active disease should receive isoniazid for 9 months if they are younger than 18 years and for at least 6 months if they are 18 years of age or older. Exposure to drug-resistant tuberculosis requires more specific therapy.
B. The child with tuberculous infection or disease may return to school or child care after drug therapy has been initiated and clinical symptoms have resolved. HIV testing should be completed for any older child or adult with tuberculosis.

References, see page 164.

Urinary Tract Infection

Urinary tract infection (UTI) is common in infants and children, and, if untreated, it can cause irreversible chronic renal failure.

Epidemiology
A. One to 2% of newborn girls and boys have UTIs. In infancy and childhood, UTI is more common in girls than in boys; 1% of school-age girls develop symptomatic infection each year.
B. Risk factors for UTI in females include sexual intercourse, sexual abuse, use of bubble bath, constipation, pinworms, and infrequent or incomplete voiding. In either sex, risk factors include ureteric reflux in a sibling, urologic abnormalities, indwelling urethral catheterization, and neurogenic bladder.
C. UTI usually is caused by bacteria that ascend up the urethra into the bladder. E coli is the most common organism associated with UTI. Other enteric bacteria include Klebsiella, Enterococcus sp, and Staphylococcus saprophyticus.

Clinical evaluation
A. In prepubertal children, UTI usually does not cause frequency, dysuria, or urgency.
B. In the newborn, signs of UTI may include late-onset jaundice, hypothermia, signs of sepsis, failure to thrive, vomiting, and fever. In infants and preschool children, additional findings include diarrhea and strong-smelling urine.
C. The school-age child may complain of frequency, dysuria, urgency, or vomiting.
D. Physical examination
   1. The growth curve should be reviewed because children who have frequent UTIs may have a decreased rate of growth.
   2. Chronic renal failure secondary to UTIs may cause hypertension. The abdominal examination may reveal tenderness, or a mass may indicate an enlarged bladder or obstructed urinary tract.
   3. Signs of vaginitis, labial adhesions, local irritation, or sexual activity/abuse should be sought. The urinary stream should be evaluated in males. A tight phimosis in an uncircumcised male infant may predispose to UTI. A rectal examination may detect masses or poor sphincter tone, indicative of neurogenic bladder.

Signs and Symptoms of UTI In Children		
Newborns	**Infants and Preschoolers**	**School-Age Children**
Jaundice	Diarrhea	Vomiting
Hypothermia	Failure to thrive	Fever
Sepsis	Vomiting	Strong-smelling urine
Failure to thrive	Fever	Abdominal pain
Vomiting	Strong-smelling urine	Frequency
Fever		Dysuria
		Urgency
		Enuresis

III. **Laboratory evaluation**
   A. **For children who have moderate-to-severe symptoms** (eg, fever, vomiting, failure to thrive, signs of sepsis), the urine specimen should be collected by catheter or suprapubic aspiration.
      1. **Bag urine specimens** are always contaminated and are not recommended for symptomatic patients. Bag urine specimens are useful only when negative.
      2. **Urinalysis.** Urine is examined by dipstick and microscopic analysis. The nitrate test is more specific for UTI than leukocyte esterase. Centrifuged urine is examined for white blood cells or bacteria.
      3. **Pyuria.** >10 WBC/mm^3 detected by microscopic analysis of an uncentrifuged specimen combined with a Gram stain analysis showing the presence of bacteria is associated with a positive urine culture in 90%.
   B. **In children who have mild symptoms,** a clean-catch urine specimen should be tested by dipstick urinalysis. If the nitrite test is negative, urine microscopy is performed; if microscopy is negative, the specimen should be cultured.

Culture Criteria for Significant Bacteriuria	
Method	**Colony Count**
Suprapubic aspiration	Any bacteria
Urethral catheterization	>10,000 cfu/mL
Best catch	$\geq$50,000 cfu/mL

IV. **Management**
   A. Patients who have severe symptoms should be treated initially with two parenteral antibiotics that provide coverage for both gram-positive and gram-negative organisms.
   B. For children whose infections are mild, a single oral antibiotic to which the patient has not been exposed recently is prescribed.

Antibiotic Therapy for Urinary Tract Infections with Severe Symptoms

Agent	Dosage (mg/kg/day)
Neonate	
Ampicillin and Gentamicin	7.5 mg/kg/day IV/IM q8h 100 mg/kg/day IV/IM q6h
Older Child	
Ceftriaxone (Rocephin)	50 mg /kg/day (IM, IV) q24h
Cefotaxime (Claforan)	100 mg /kg/day (IV) q6-8h
Ampicillin/sulbactam (Unasyn)	100-200 mg of ampicillin/kg/day q6h
Gentamicin	3-7.5 mg /kg/day(IV, IM) q8h

Antibiotic Therapy for Urinary Tract Infections with Mild Symptoms

Agent	Dosage
Cefpodoxime (Vantin)	10 mg/kg/day PO q12h [susp: 50 mg/5 mL, 100 mg/5 mL; tabs: 100 mg, 200 mg]
Cefprozil (Cefzil)	30 mg/kg/day PO q12h [susp: 125 mg/5 mL, 250 mg/5 mL; tabs: 250, 500 mg]
Cefixime (Suprax)	8 mg/kg/d PO qd-bid [susp: 100 mg/5 mL, tab: 200,400 mg]
Cefuroxime (Ceftin)	125-500 mg PO q12h [125, 250, 500 mg]
Amoxicillin/clavulanate (Augmentin)	40 mg of amoxicillin kg/day PO q8h [susp: amoxicillin 125 mg/clavulanate/5 mL; tab: amoxicillin 250 mg/clavulanate; amoxicillin 500 mg/clavulanate]
Trimethoprim/sulfamethoxazole (Bactrim)	6-12 mg/kg/day (trimethoprim) q12h [susp: trimethoprim 40 mg/sulfamethoxazole 200 mg/5 mL]

C. A urine culture should be repeated early in the course of treatment if symptoms persist.

D. Most patients are treated for 10 days; those treated parenterally can be switched to oral therapy when symptoms have resolved and antimicrobial susceptibilities are known.

E. **Follow-up screening.** After the first infection is treated successfully, follow-up screening for UTI is indicated at 1 month, 3 months, 6 months, 12 months, and yearly. Home nitrite testing on first-morning urine specimens is an accurate method for follow-up.

. **Imaging studies**
A. Imaging studies are recommended in the following patients:

       1. UTI in a male.
       2. UTI in an infant.
       3. Pyelonephritis in a female.
       4. Recurrent UTI in a female.
   B. Early renal ultrasonography should be obtained to look for evidence of urina‹ tract obstruction. If results show abnormalities, radioactive renal scanning useful for defining renal anatomy more precisely.
   C. A voiding cystourethrogram should be performed to define urethral and bladd‹ anatomy. Children who have UTI with simple reflux usually can be observe‹ as long as recurrent infection is prevented.

VI. Prevention of recurrent urinary tract infection
   A. Uncircumcised males with phimosis may benefit from circumcision. Front-to-ba‹ wiping should be encouraged, bubble baths should be eliminated, showers encourage‹ and pinworms should be treated.
   B. A high fluid intake and a frequent voiding schedule is recommended. Constipatio‹ should be identified and treated. Patients with postcoital UTI should void aft‹ intercourse and perhaps take antimicrobial prophylaxis after intercourse.
   C. Patients with significant ureteral reflux ≥grade 1, and those with frequent recurrenc‹ require long-term (6 months to 2 years) prophylaxis, which can be achieved wi‹ sulfisoxazole (Gantrisin), 30 mg/kg qhs.

References, see page 164.

Viral Laryngotracheitis (Croup)

Acute laryngotracheitis (viral croup) is the most common infectious cause of acute upp‹ airway obstruction in pediatrics, causing 90% of cases. The disease is usually self-limite‹ Children in the 1- to 2-year-old age group are most commonly affected. Viral cro‹ affects 3-5% of all children each year. Croup is most common from the late fall to ea‹ spring, although cases may occur throughout the year.

I. Clinical evaluation of upper airway obstruction and stridor
   A. Stridor is the most common presenting feature of all causes of acute upper airw‹ obstruction. It is a harsh sound that results from air movement through a partial‹ obstructed upper airway.
      1. Supraglottic disorders, such as epiglottitis, cause quiet, wet stridor, a muffle‹ voice, dysphagia and a preference for sitting upright.
      2. Subglottic lesions, such as croup, cause loud stridor accompanied by a hoars‹ voice and barky cough.
   B. Patient age
      1. Upper airway obstruction in school age and older children tends to be cause‹ by severe tonsillitis or peritonsillar abscesses.
      2. From infancy to 2 years of age, viral croup and retropharyngeal abscess a‹ the most common causes of upper airway obstruction.
   C. Mode of onset
      1. Gradual onset of symptoms, usually preceded by upper respiratory infecti‹ symptoms, suggests viral croup, severe tonsillitis or retropharyngeal absces‹
      2. Very acute onset of symptoms suggests epiglottitis.
      3. A history of a choking episode or intermittent respiratory distress sugges‹ a foreign body inhalation.
      4. Facial edema and urticaria suggests angioedema.
   D. Emergency management of upper airway obstruction
      1. Maintaining an adequate airway takes precedence over other diagnostic interventio‹

If a supraglottic disorder is suspected, a person skilled at intubation must accompany the child at all times.

2. Patients with suspected epiglottitis, severe respiratory distress from an obstruction, or suspected foreign body inhalation should be taken to the operating room for direct laryngoscopic visualization and possible intubation.

Causes of Upper Airway Obstruction in Children

Supraglottic Infectious Disorders
Epiglottitis
Peritonsillar abscess
Retropharyngeal abscess
Severe tonsillitis

Subglottic Infectious Disorders
Croup (viral laryngotracheitis)
Spasmodic croup
Bacterial tracheitis

Non-Infectious Causes
Angioedema
Foreign body aspiration
Congenital obstruction
Neoplasms
External trauma to neck

Characteristics of selected causes of Upper Airway Obstruction

	Epiglottitis	Laryngotra-cheobronchitis (Croup)	Bacterial Tracheitis	Foreign Body Aspiration
History				
Incidence in children presenting with stridor	8%	88%	2%	2%
Onset	Rapid, 4-12 hours	Prodrome, 1-7 days	Prodrome, 3 days, then 10 hours	Acute or chronic
Age	1-6 years	3 mo-3 years	3 mo-2 years	Any
Season	None	October-May	None	None
Etiology	Haemophilus influenza	Parainfluenza viruses	Staphylococcus	Many
Pathology	Inflammatory edema of epiglottis and supraglottitis	Edema and inflammation of trachea and bronchial tree	Tracheal-bronchial edema, necrotic debris	Localized tracheitis
Signs and Symptoms				
Dysphagia	Yes	No	No	Rare

	Epiglottitis	Laryngotra-cheobronchitis (Croup)	Bacterial Tracheitis	Foreign Body Aspiration
Difficulty swallowing	Yes	No	Rare	No
Drooling	Yes	No	Rare	No
Stridor	Inspiratory	Inspiratory and expiratory	Inspiratory	Variable
Voice	Muffled	Hoarse	Normal	Variable
Cough	No	Barking	Variable	Yes
Temperature	Markedly elevated	Minimally elevated	Moderate	Normal
Heart rate	Increased early	Increased late	Proportional to fever	Normal
Position	Erect, anxious, "air hungry," supine position exacerbates	No effect on air-way obstruction	No effect	No effect
Respiratory rate	Increased early	Increased late	Normal	Increased if bron-chial obstruction present

Differentiation of Epiglottitis from Viral Laryngotracheitis		
Clinical Feature	Epiglottitis	Viral Croup
Retractions	present	present
Wheezing	absent	occasionally present
Cyanosis	present	present in severe cases
"Toxicity"	present	absent
Preference for sitting	yes	no

II. **Epidemiology and etiology of viral laryngotracheitis (Croup)**
   A. **Parainfluenza virus type 1** causes 40% of all cases of laryngotracheitis. Parainfluenza type 3, respiratory syncytial virus (RSV), parainfluenza type 2, and rhinovirus may also cause croup.
   B. RSV commonly affects infants younger than 12 months of age, causing wheezing and stridor. Influenza viruses A and B and mycoplasma have been implicated in patients older than 5 years.
III. **Clinical manifestations**
   A. Viral croup begins gradually with a 1-2 day prodrome, resembling an upper respiratory infection. Subglottic edema and inflammation of the larynx, trachea, and bronchi eventually develop.
   B. Low-grade fever and nocturnal exacerbation of cough are common. As airway obstruction increases retractions, develop, restlessness, anxiety, tachycardia,

and tachypnea may occur.

   C. Cyanosis is a late sign. Severe obstruction leads to respiratory muscle exhaustion, hypoxemia, carbon dioxide accumulation, and respiratory acidosis. Stridor becomes less apparent as muscle fatigue worsens.

   D. Ten percent of croup patients have severe respiratory compromise requiring hospital admission, and 3% of those children need airway support.

IV. **Laboratory evaluation**. The diagnosis of viral croup is based primarily on the history and clinical findings. When the diagnosis is uncertain or the patient requires hospitalization, x-rays can be helpful. The posteroanterior neck radiograph of a patient with viral croup shows symmetrical narrowing of the subglottic space ("steeple sign").

V. **Inpatient treatment of laryngotracheitis**

   A. The majority of patients who have croup do not require hospitalization.

   B. **Indications for hospitalization**

      1. Dusky or cyanotic skin color.
      2. Decreased air entry on auscultation.
      3. Severe stridor.
      4. Significant retractions.
      5. Agitation, restlessness, or obtundation.

   C. Signs that indicate the need for an artificial airway include decreased respiratory effort and decreased level of consciousness. Pulse oximetry may aid in assessing the severity of respiratory compromise.

   D. All patients suspected of having viral croup should be given humidified air. Hypoxic or cyanotic patients require oxygen via mask and may require intubation. Oral hydration is essential to help loosen secretions; however, intravenous hydration may become necessary in the very ill child.

   E. **Racemic epinephrine** has alpha-adrenergic properties, which decrease subglottic inflammation and edema. Racemic epinephrine is administered as 0.5 mL of a 2.25% solution, diluted with 3.5 mL of saline (1:8) by nebulization. It is given every 20-30 minutes for severe croup, and it is given every 4-6 hours for moderate croup.

   F. **Corticosteroids** reduce subglottic edema and inflammation. **Dexamethasone** (0.6 mg/kg IM) given one time early in the course of croup results in a shorter hospital stay and reduces cough and dyspnea. Patients who do not require hospitalization should not receive steroids.

   G. **Acetaminophen** decreases fever and oxygen consumption in the febrile patient with croup.

   H. Patients with mild viral croup usually are not admitted to the hospital and can be treated safely at home. Vaporizers, oral fluids, and antipyretics are the mainstays of home therapy. The prognosis for croup is good; however, a subset of children

who have croup will later be identified as having asthma.
References, see page 164.

Pelvic Inflammatory Disease

Pelvic inflammatory disease (PID) is an acute infection of the upper genital tract in women, involving any or all of the uterus, oviducts, and ovaries. PID is a community-acquired infection initiated by a sexually transmitted agent. Pelvic inflammatory disease accounts for approximately 2.5 million outpatient visits and 200,000 hospitalizations annually.

I. **Clinical evaluation**
   A. Lower abdominal pain is the cardinal presenting symptom in women with PID, although the character of the pain may be quite subtle. The onset of pain during or shortly after menses is particularly suggestive. The abdominal pain is usually bilateral and rarely of more than two weeks' duration.
   B. Abnormal uterine bleeding occurs in one-third or more of patients with PID. New vaginal discharge, urethritis, proctitis, fever, and chills can be associated signs.
   C. Risk factors for PID:
      1. Age less than 35 years
      2. Nonbarrier contraception
      3. New, multiple, or symptomatic sexual partners
      4. Previous episode of PID
      5. Oral contraception
      6. African-American ethnicity

II. **Physical examination**
   A. Only one-half of patients with PID have fever. Abdominal examination reveals diffuse tenderness greatest in the lower quadrants, which may or may not be symmetrical. Rebound tenderness and decreased bowel sounds are common. Tenderness in the right upper quadrant does not exclude PID, because approximately 10 percent of these patients have perihepatitis (Fitz-Hugh Curtis syndrome).
   B. Purulent endocervical discharge and/or acute cervical motion and adnexal tenderness by bimanual examination is strongly suggestive of PID. Rectovaginal examination should reveal the uterine adnexal tenderness.

III. **Diagnosis**
   A. **Diagnostic criteria and guidelines**. The index of suspicion for the clinical diagnosis of PID should be high, especially in adolescent women.
   B. The CDC has recommended minimum criteria required for empiric treatment of PID. These major determinants include lower abdominal tenderness, adnexal tenderness, and cervical motion tenderness. Minor determinants (ie, signs that may increase the suspicion of PID) include:
      1. Fever (oral temperature >101°F; >38.3°C)
      2. Vaginal discharge
      3. Documented STD
      4. Erythrocyte sedimentation rate (ESR)
      5. C-reactive protein
      6. Systemic signs
      7. Dyspareunia
   C. **Empiric treatment for pelvic inflammatory disease is recommended when:**
      1. The examination suggests PID
      2. Demographics (risk factors) are consistent with PID
      3. Pregnancy test is negative

Laboratory Evaluation for Pelvic Inflammatory Disease

- Pregnancy test
- Microscopic exam of vaginal discharge in saline
- Complete blood counts
- Tests for chlamydia and gonococcus
- Urinalysis
- Fecal occult blood test
- C-reactive protein(optional)

IV. Diagnostic testing

A. Laboratory testing for patients suspected of having PID always begins with a pregnancy test to rule out ectopic pregnancy and complications of an intrauterine pregnancy. A urinalysis and a stool for occult blood should be obtained because abnormalities in either reduce the probability of PID. Blood counts have limited value. Fewer than one-half of PID patients exhibit leukocytosis.

B. Gram stain and microscopic examination of vaginal discharge may provide useful information. If a cervical Gram stain is positive for Gram-negative intracellular diplococci, the probability of PID greatly increases; if negative, it is of little use.

C. Increased white blood cells (WBC) in vaginal fluid may be the most sensitive single laboratory test for PID (78 percent for $\geq$3 WBC per high power field. However, the specificity is only 39 percent.

D. Recommended laboratory tests:
1. Pregnancy test
2. Microscopic exam of vaginal discharge in saline
3. Complete blood counts
4. Tests for chlamydia and gonococcus
5. Urinalysis
6. Fecal occult blood test
7. C-reactive protein(optional)

E. Ultrasound imaging is reserved for acutely ill patients with PID in whom a pelvic abscess is a consideration.

V. Recommendations

A. Health care providers should maintain a low threshold for the diagnosis of PID, and sexually active young women with lower abdominal, adnexal, and cervical motion tenderness should receive empiric treatment. The specificity of these clinical criteria can be enhanced by the presence of fever, abnormal cervical/vaginal discharge, elevated ESR and/or serum C-reactive protein, and the demonstration of cervical gonorrhea or chlamydia infection.

B. If clinical findings (epidemiologic, symptomatic, and physical examination) suggest PID empiric treatment should be initiated.

Differential Diagnosis of Pelvic Inflammatory Disease

Appendicitis	Irritable bowel syndrome
Ectopic pregnancy	Somatization
Hemorrhagic ovarian cyst	Gastroenteritis
Ovarian torsion	Cholecystitis
Endometriosis	Nephrolithiasis
Urinary tract Infection	

VI. Treatment of pelvic inflammatory disease

A. The two most important initiators of PID, Neisseria gonorrhoeae and Chlamydia trachomatis, must be treated, but coverage should also be provided for groups A and B streptococci, Gram negative enteric bacilli (Escherichia coli, Klebsiella spp., and Proteus spp.), and anaerobes.

B. **Outpatient therapy**

   1. For outpatient therapy, the CDC recommends either oral ofloxacin (Floxin, 400 mg twice daily) or levofloxacin (Levaquin, 500 mg once daily) with or without metronidazole (Flagyl, 500 mg twice daily) for 14 days. An alternative is an initial single dose of ceftriaxone (Rocephin, 250 mg IM), cefoxitin (Mefoxin, 2 g IM plus probenecid 1 g orally), or another parenteral third-generation cephalosporin, followed by doxycycline (100 mg orally twice daily) with or without metronidazole for 14 days. Quinolones are not recommended to treat gonorrhea acquired in California or Hawaii. If the patient may have acquired the disease in Asia, Hawaii, or California, cefixime or ceftriaxone should be used.

   2. Another alternative is azithromycin (Zithromax, 1 g PO for Chlamydia coverage) and amoxicillin-clavulanate (Amoxicillin, 875 mg PO) once by directly observed therapy, followed by amoxicillin-clavulanate (Amoxicillin, 875 mg PO BID) for 7 to 10 days.

C. **Inpatient therapy**

   1. For inpatient treatment, the CDC suggests either of the following regimens:
      a. **Cefotetan (Cefotan)**, 2 g IV Q12h, or cefoxitin (Mefoxin, 2 g IV Q6h) plus doxycycline (100 mg IV or PO Q12h)
      b. **Clindamycin (Cleocin)**, 900 mg IV Q8h, plus gentamicin (1-1.5 mg/kg IV q8h)

   2. Alternative regimens:
      a. **Ofloxacin (Floxin)**, 400 mg IV Q12h or levofloxacin (Levaquin, 500 mg IV QD) with or without metronidazole (Flagyl, 500 mg IV Q8h). Quinolones are not recommended to treat gonorrhea acquired in California or Hawaii. If the patient may have acquired the disease in Asia, Hawaii, or California, cefixime or ceftriaxone should be used.
      b. **Ampicillin-sulbactam (Unasyn)**, 3 g IV Q6h plus doxycycline (100 mg IV or PO Q12h)

   3. Parenteral administration of antibiotics should be continued for 24 hours after clinical response, followed by doxycycline (100 mg PO BID) or clindamycin (Cleocin, 450 mg PO QID) for a total of 14 days.

   4. **The following regimen may also be used: Levofloxacin (Levaquin)**, 500 mg IV Q24h, plus metronidazole (Flagyl, 500 mg IV Q8h). With this regimen, azithromycin (Zithromax, 1 g PO once) should be given as soon as the patient is tolerating oral intake. Parenteral therapy is continued until the pelvic tenderness on bimanual examination is mild or absent.

D. **Annual screening** is recommended for all sexually active women under age 25 and for women over 25 if they have new or multiple sexual partners. A retest for chlamydia should be completed in 3 to 4 months after chlamydia treatment because of high rates of reinfection.

E. **Additional evaluation:**

   1. Serology for the human immunodeficiency virus (HIV)
   2. Papanicolaou smear
   3. Hepatitis B surface antigen determination and initiation of the vaccine series for patients who are antigen negative and unvaccinated
   4. Hepatitis C virus serology
   5. Serologic tests for syphilis

References, see page 164.

Gastrointestinal Disorders

Acute Abdominal Pain

The evaluation of abdominal pain in children is problematic because the pain is often difficult to localize, and the history in children is often nonspecific.

I. **Localization of abdominal pain**
   A. **Generalized pain** in the epigastrium usually comes from the stomach, duodenum, or the pancreas.
   B. **Periumbilical pain** usually originates in small bowel and colon or spleen.
   C. **Parietal pain,** caused by inflammation, is usually well localized.
   D. **Referred abdominal pain** occurs when poorly localized visceral pain is felt at a distant location.
      1. **Pancreatitis, cholecystitis, liver abscess,** or a splenic hemorrhage cause diaphragmatic irritation, which is referred to the ipsilateral neck and shoulders.
      2. **Intraabdominal fluid** may cause shoulder pain on reclining.
      3. **Gallbladder pain** may be felt in the lower back or infrascapular area.
      4. **Pancreatic pain** often is referred to the posterior flank.
      5. **Ureterolithiasis** often presents as pain radiating toward the ipsilateral groin.
      6. **Rectal or gynecological pain** often is perceived as sacral pain.
      7. **Right lower lobe pneumonia** may be perceived as right upper quadrant abdominal pain.

II. **Clinical evaluation**
   A. **History** should include the quality, timing, and type of abdominal pain.
      1. **Pain of sudden onset** often denotes colic, perforation or acute ischemia caused by torsion or volvulus.
      2. **Slower onset** of pain suggests inflammatory conditions, such as appendicitis, pancreatitis, or cholecystitis.
   B. **Colic** results from spasms of a hollow viscus organ secondary to an obstruction. It is characterized by severe, intermittent cramping, followed by intervals when the pain is less intense. Colic pain usually originates from the biliary tree, pancreatic duct, gastrointestinal tract, urinary system, or uterus and tubes.
   C. **Inflammatory pain** is caused by peritoneal irritation, and the patient presents quietly without much motion and appears ill. The pain is initially less severe and is exacerbated by movement.
   D. **Vomiting.** Usually abdominal pain will precede vomiting. The interval between abdominal pain and vomiting is shorter when associated with colic. Delayed vomiting for many hours is often associated with distal bowel obstruction or ileus secondary to peritonitis.
   E. **Diarrhea.** Mild diarrhea with the onset of abdominal pain suggests acute gastroenteritis or early appendicitis. Delayed onset of diarrhea may indicate a perforated appendicitis, with the inflamed mass causing irritation of the sigmoid colon.
   F. **Physical examination**
      1. The abdomen should be observed, auscultated, and palpated for distention, localized tenderness, masses, and peritonitis. The groin must be examined to exclude an incarcerated hernia or ovary, or torsion of an ovary or testicle.
      2. **Rectal examination**
         a. **Gross blood in the stool** suggests ectopic gastric mucosa, Meckel's diverticula, or polyps.

b. **Blood and mucus** (currant jelly stool) suggests inflammatory bowel disease or intussusception.

c. **Melena** suggests upper gastrointestinal bleeding, necessitating gastric aspiration for blood.

d. **Tests for occult blood** in the stool should be performed.

3. **Pelvic examinations** are mandatory for postmenarchal and/or sexually active female patients. The rectal examination may also be used to evaluate the cervix, uterus, adnexa, and pelvic masses.

4. **Fever**

a. Thoracic disease (eg, pneumonia) may be the cause of abdominal pain associated with fever.

b. Costovertebral angle tenderness with fever suggests pyelonephritis or a high retrocecal appendicitis.

III. Appendicitis

A. **Fever, vomiting, irritability, lethargy with right lower quadrant (RLQ) tenderness and guarding** are diagnostic of appendicitis in the very young patient until proven otherwise. A mass may be felt on rectal exam in 2-7% of younger patients with appendicitis.

B. A WBC >15,000 supports the diagnosis. An ultrasound of the appendix may be useful.

C. **Children older than 2 years old** present with a perforated appendix about 30-60% of the time. This incidence declines as the age of the child increases.

IV. Intussusception

A. Intussusception is the most common cause of bowel obstruction between 2 months and 5 years of age. The most vulnerable age group is 4-10 months old, but children up to 7 years old may be at risk.

B. Intussusception is characterized by vomiting, colicky abdominal pain (85%) with drawing up of the legs, and currant jelly stools (60%). Fever is common.

C. The abdomen may be soft and nontender between episodes of colicky pain, but eventually it becomes distended. A sausage-shaped mass in the right upper quadrant (RUQ) may be palpable.

D. **Abdominal x-ray.** The leading edge of the intussusception is usually outlined with air, which will establish the diagnosis. Often there are radiographic signs of bowel obstruction. When the plain abdominal x-ray is normal, intussusception cannot be excluded without a barium enema.

E. **Treatment** consists of radiologic reduction, which is effective in 80-90%. Radiographic reduction is contraindicated if there is peritoneal irritation or toxicity.

V. Midgut volvulus

A. Midgut volvulus results from the improper rotation and fixation of the duodenum and colon (malrotation). Obstruction of the superior mesenteric artery may cause ischemic necrosis of the gut, which may be fatal.

B. Infants in the first month constitute the majority of the cases. Symptoms usually begin about 5 days before diagnosis. The first sign of volvulus is bilious vomiting, followed by abdominal distention and GI bleeding. Peritonitis, hypovolemia, and shock may follow.

C. **Abdominal x-ray** reveals a classic double bubble caused by duodenal obstruction. Pneumatosis intestinalis or distal bowel obstruction may also be apparent.

D. Infants with rapid deterioration and obstructed loops of bowel require immediate surgery. If the infant is not critically ill, an UGI series with water-soluble, non-ionic, isoosmolar contrast will confirm midgut volvulus. If malrotation or volvulus (beak, spiral or corkscrew sign) is found, an immediate laparotomy is necessary.

VI. Gallbladder disease

A. **Cholecystitis** in children occurs most commonly in the adolescent female, but it may affect infants who are only a few weeks of age. Cholecystitis is suggested by RUQ pain, back pain, or epigastric pain, radiating to the right subscapular area, bilious vomiting, fever, RUQ tenderness, and a RUQ mass. Jaundice is present in 25-55%, usually in association with hemolytic disease.

B. Ultrasonography delineates gallstones and is the study of choice to screen for gallbladder disease.

C. Radioisotopic scanning evaluates biliary and gallbladder function.

VII. Ectopic pregnancy

A. Ectopic pregnancy must be considered in any postmenarchal, sexually active adolescent with abdominal pain. It is uncommon and usually seen in late adolescence. Ectopic pregnancy occurs in 0.5-3% of all pregnancies.

B. Signs of ectopic pregnancy include abdominal pain in any location, vaginal bleeding, and/or amenorrhea. Nausea and vomiting, other symptoms of pregnancy, and lightheadedness may also be present.

C. Abdominal, adnexal, and/or cervical tenderness are often found on pelvic examination, but occasionally abdominal tenderness is absent. The cervix may be soft (Godell's sign) and bluish in color (Chadwick's sign). The examination may reveal adnexal fullness and uterine enlargement.

D. Evaluation includes a pregnancy test and ultrasound. Treatment consists of removal of the ectopic pregnancy by laparoscopy or exploratory laparotomy.

VIII. Gonadal pain in males

A. In males with lower abdominal pain, the scrotum and its contents must be examined. Testicular torsion is a surgical emergency and must be treated within 6 hours of the onset of the pain to save the testicle.

B. Testicular torsion may present as lower abdominal pain, which may be associated with recent trauma or cold. The gonad is tender and elevated in the scrotum, with a transverse orientation. Although testicular torsion may occur at any age, it usually occurs in adolescent males at puberty or shortly afterwards.

IX. Gonadal pain in females

A. The leading causes of gonadal pain in females are ovarian cysts and torsion of uterine adnexal structures.

B. Ovarian cysts are responsible for 25% of childhood ovarian tumors, most commonly in adolescents. Bleeding into the cyst or cystic rupture causes pain, which usually subsides within 12-24 hours. Ultrasound may show pelvic fluid and the cyst.

C. Torsion of uterine adnexal structures

1. Torsion is associated with unilateral, sudden, severe pain with nausea and vomiting. The patient may also have subacute or chronic symptoms, with intermittent pain for days. The pain is usually diffuse and periumbilical in younger patients, but in older children and adolescents, the pain may radiate initially to the anterior thigh or ipsilateral groin.

2. Fever and leucocytosis are usually present. Physical exam may reveal muscle rigidity and fixation of the mass on pelvic examination.

3. Ultrasound will identify the mass accurately. Surgical exploration may sometimes salvage the ovary. Malignant neoplasms may cause torsion in 35% of cases.

X. Meckel diverticulum

A. Meckel diverticulum are present in 2% of the population. It presents as a tender left lower quadrant mass, associated with blood in the stool.

B. Vague abdominal pain with hemoccult positive stools suggests a Meckel diverticulum. Bleeding is seen in 35-40% of childhood cases. A technetium nuclear scan may confirm the diagnosis.

References, see page 164.

Recurrent Abdominal Pain

Recurrent abdominal pain (RAP) includes any child or adolescent who has recurrent abdominal pain for which the family seeks medical attention and explanation. More than 90% of the time a "disease" will not be defined and the family will be left with a "functional" explanation.

I. Epidemiology

A. RAP occurs in 10-15% of children between the ages of 4 and 16 years. About 13-17% of adolescents experience weekly pain. The overall incidence appears to peak at 10 to 12 years. RAP is rare among children younger than 5 years of age.

Differential Diagnosis of Recurrent Abdominal Pain

- Functional abdominal pain
- Fecal impaction
- Parasitic infection
- Partial small bowel obstruction
  - Crohn disease
  - Malrotation with or without volvulus
  - Intussusception
  - Postsurgical adhesions
  - Small bowel lymphoma
  - Infection (tuberculosis, Yersinia)
  - Eosinophilic gastroenteritis
  - Angioneurotic edema
- Ureteropelvic junction obstruction
- Appendiceal colic

- Dysmenorrhea
  - Endometriosis
  - Ectopic pregnancy
  - Adhesions from pelvic inflammatory disease
- Cystic teratoma of ovary
- Musculoskeletal disorders
  - Muscle pain
  - Linea alba hernia
  - Discitis
- Vascular disorders
  - Mesenteric thrombosis
  - Polyarteritis nodosa
- Abdominal migraine
- Acute intermittent porphyria
- Psychiatric disorders

Diagnostic Criteria for Functional Abdominal Pain

- Chronicity
- Compatible age range, age of onset
- Characteristic features of abdominal pain
- Evidence of physical or psychological stressful stimuli
- Environmental reinforcement of pain behavior
- Normal physical examination (including rectal examination and stool guaiac)
- Normal laboratory evaluation (CBC, sedimentation rate, urinalysis, urine culture, stool ova and parasites)

II. Clinical Aspects

A. **Functional abdominal pain.** The majority of children who have RAP are considered to have a functional etiology, and an organic etiology cannot be found. The pain occurs in episodes that are periumbilical, self-limited, unrelated to meals or activities, and rarely if ever sufficient to awaken the child from sleep. The growth pattern and findings on the physical examination are normal. The degree of interference with normal activities and school attendance are out of proportion to the frequency and severity of the episodes.

B. **Irritable bowel syndrome.** Some children who have RAP manifest characteristics of irritable bowel syndrome (IBS). The criteria for making this diagnosis are: 1) abdominal pain relieved by defecation, 2) more frequent stools at the onset of the pain, 3) altered stool form (hard or loose or watery), 4) passage of mucus, and 5) associated bloating or abdominal distension.

C. **Constipation**. The most common causes of constipation in children are inadequate intake of fruits, vegetables and higher-fiber foods, and an unwillingness to evacuate the bowels. The child goes days between bowel movements and the stool is bulky and hard. Findings on abdominal and rectal examinations may confirm the diagnosis; a plain abdominal radiograph may be needed.

D. **Inflammatory bowel disease.** Ulcerative colitis may present with abdominal pain, hematochezia and tenesmus. Crohn disease may cause abdominal pain, diarrhea, lethargy, growth and pubertal delay, and oral, joint, and perirectal involvement. Endoscopy will confirm the diagnosis.

E. **Lactose intolerance**. Asian, Jewish, Mediterranean, and African-American persons are predisposed to lactase deficiency. Lactose ingestion will cause bloating, loose stools, and cramping abdominal pain. The diagnosis is made by breath hydrogen testing or a therapeutic trial of restriction of milk products.

F. **Helicobacter pylori-associated peptic ulcer disease** should be suspected when abdominal pain is primarily epigastric; when it awakens the child from sleep; and when it is associated with anorexia, nausea, recurrent vomiting, anemia, or gastrointestinal bleeding. Peptic ulcer disease is very uncommon is children; therefore, testing for H pylori should not be part of the preliminary evaluation of a child who has RAP.

G. **Nonulcer dyspepsia** is a symptom complex of epigastric pain, bloating, and discomfort accompanied by negative endoscopic and biopsy findings.

H. **Abdominal migraine** usually is recognized when episodes of paroxysmal abdominal pain occur in association with nausea and vomiting, sometimes with associated headache. A strong family history of migraine is usually present.

I. **Infestation/infection**. Infection with Yersinia enterocolitica and giardia can cause diarrhea associated with abdominal cramps and pain, but diarrhea usually is the predominant complaint.

J. **Gynecologic conditions**. Early menarche, endometriosis, pelvic inflammatory disease, and ovarian cyst may cause RAP. These causes can be diagnosed by ultrasonographic examination.

K. **Physical and sexual abuse** may cause RAP, and sensitive history taking is required to elucidate its possible role.

III. **Clinical assessment**

A. The history should assess the location, nature, frequency of the pain, and associated symptoms. The relationship of the pain to school and social/family stressors is important. Review of systems should cover the child's diet, bowel habits, sleep patterns, and context in which the pain occurs.

B. The degree to which the pain interferes with the child's activities should be defined. Family function, school performance, anxiety, depression, or social maladjustment should be assessed. Medication use should be assessed.

"Red Flags" on History of Recurrent Abdominal Pain

- Localization of the pain away from the umbilicus
- Pain associated with change in bowel habits, particularly diarrhea, constipation, or nocturnal bowel movements
- Pain associated with night wakening
- Repetitive emesis, especially if bilious
- Constitutional symptoms, such as recurrent fever, loss of appetite or energy
- RAP occurring in a child younger than 4 years of age

C. **Physical Examination.** Height and weight should be recorded and compared to previous growth data. The abdomen should be examined gently and thoroughly while observing the child's response to palpation. The perianal area should be examined for fissures, skin tags, or signs of sexual abuse. A rectal examination is not routinely performed.

"Red Flags" on Physical Examination for Recurrent Abdominal Pain

- Loss of weight or decline in height velocity
- Organomegaly
- Localized abdominal tenderness, particularly removed from the umbilicus
- Perirectal abnormalities (eg, fissures, ulceration, or skin tags)
- Joint swelling, redness, or heat
- Ventral hernias of the abdominal wall

IV. **Investigations**
   A. **Laboratory investigations** should usually be limited to a complete blood count, urinalysis, and examination of a stool specimen for occult blood. In the presence of diarrhea, a stool for enteric culture and ova and parasite examination is indicated.
   B. **Radiography.** A single view of the abdomen can be useful to confirm constipation.
   C. **Abdominal ultrasonography** can be valuable when obstructive uropathy hydronephrosis, ovarian cysts, or gall bladder disorders are suspected. Enteric duplication also may be revealed by ultrasonography. Ultrasound is appropriate when the pain is lateralized, when there are abnormalities on urinalysis, or when the pain localizes to the lower quadrants in a female.
   D. **Erythrocyte sedimentation rate**, serum protein and albumin levels, and stool for occult blood should be obtained. If IBD is a possible diagnosis. Endoscopy and biopsy will confirm the diagnosis. Upper gastrointestinal endoscopy with biopsies will confirm the diagnosis when the pattern of pain strongly suggests peptic ulcer disease.

V. **Management**
   A. **Functional recurrent abdominal pain** will be the diagnosis in the majority of cases. The parents should maintain a sympathetic attitude that acknowledges the pain but encourages continued activities and school attendance. Parents should refrain from questioning the child about the pain if the child is not complaining. A trial of increasing fiber by dietary modification may be useful.
   B. **Psychogenic pain** may respond to the intervention of a psychologist or psychiatrist
   C. **Constipation** requires treatment with regular stool softeners, preceded by an enema.
   D. **Lactose malabsorption.** A lactose-free diet for several weeks with lactase-treated milk should be tried. Ice cream and cheese should be avoided.
   E. **Enteric infections or infestations** require treatment with appropriate medications. Abdominal migraine may warrant a trial of migraine prophylaxis. Prophylactic pizotifen cyproheptadine, propranolol, or amitriptyline could be considered.

References, see page 164.

Chronic Nonspecific Diarrhea

iarrhea is considered chronic when it persists for longer than 3 weeks. Chronic nonspecific iarrhea (CNSD) presents in toddlers between 18 months and 3 years of age, with frequent, arge, watery stools in the absence of physical or laboratory signs of malabsorption r infection and without effect on growth or development. Children have 3 to 6 large, atery bowel movements daily. The diarrhea spontaneously resolves in 90% of children y 40 months of age.

Pathogenesis
A. Factors causing CNSD
1. Excess fluid intake
2. Carbohydrate malabsorption from excessive juice ingestion
3. Disordered intestinal motility
4. Excessive fecal bile acids
5. Low fat intake
B. CNSD occurs when fluid intake exceeds the absorptive capacity of the intestinal tract. Malabsorption of carbohydrates (sucrose, fructose, sorbitol) in fruit juices contributes to CNSD.
C. CNSD presents between 18 months and 3 years, with 3-6 large, loose, watery stools per day for more than 3 weeks.
D. Stooling is most frequent in the morning and does not occur during sleep. There is an absence of nausea, vomiting, abdominal pain, flatulence, blood, fever, anorexia, weight loss, or poor growth.

I. Clinical evaluation of chronic nonspecific diarrhea
A. The current number and type of stools should be determined. A diet history should determine the total calories, fat, milk and juice consumed daily, and it should assess prior trials of food elimination.
B. The timing of introduction of foods into the diet relative to the onset of diarrhea, and a 3-day diet history should be assessed. Usage of antibiotics, vitamins, iron, and medications should be sought.
C. A family history of irritable bowel syndrome, celiac disease, inflammatory bowel disease, infectious diarrhea, or food allergies should be sought.
D. Physical examination
1. Growth chart plotting of weight, height, and head circumference are essential. Children who have CNSD should continue to grow normally; deviation from the growth chart or a downward trend suggests inadequate caloric intake or a disease other than CNSD.
2. Signs of malnutrition or malabsorption include lack of subcutaneous fat, eczematoid rash (from essential fatty acid deficiency), glossitis, easy bruising, or hyporeflexia.
E. Laboratory tests
1. A fresh stool specimen is tested for neutral fat, pH and reducing substances, occult blood, and Giardia antigen. Neutral fat suggest pancreatic insufficiency.
2. Fecal pH and reducing substances will reveal carbohydrate malabsorption if the pH is less than 5.5 or if reducing substances are greater than 1+.
3. Occult fecal blood is inconsistent with CNSD unless there is a perianal rash.
4. Giardia and Cryptosporidium are common and should be excluded with 3 stool samples for ova and parasites.

Stool Evaluation		
Test	Result	Disease
pH	<5.5	Carbohydrate malabsorption
Reducing substances	>1+	
Neutral fat	>40 globules/high power field	Pancreatic insufficiency
Occult blood	Positive	Enteritis or colitis
Giardia antigen	Positive	Giardiasis
Ova and parasites	Positive	Giardiasis, cryptosporidiosis

III. **Differential diagnosis**
   A. The differential diagnosis of chronic diarrhea in the 6- to 36-month-old child include disaccharidase deficiency, protein intolerance, enteric infection, and malabsorption
   B. **Lactase deficiency**
      1. **Lactase deficiency** may cause diarrhea associated with milk ingestion.
      2. **Congenital lactase deficiency** is extremely rare and symptoms are present from birth if an infant is fed human milk or a lactose-containing formula.
      3. **Genetically acquired lactase deficiency** is common, but it usually is not symptomatic before 5 years of age.
   C. **Congenital sucrase-isomaltase deficiency** is rare, producing symptoms when sucrose-containing formula or foods are introduced.
   D. **Disaccharidase deficiency** can be confirmed by eliminating the specific carbohydrate or by breath hydrogen analysis.
   E. **Milk-induced colitis** occurs in infants younger than 1 year of age who typically appear healthy but lose blood in their stool after ingesting milk protein. Infants who have milk-induced enterocolitis are younger, less than 3 months of age. These infants may be severely ill with bloody diarrhea, hypoproteinemia, and growth failure. Children who have protein allergies tend to come from families that have allergic histories, and affected children may have eczema, allergic rhinitis, asthma.
   F. **Giardia or Cryptosporidium enteric infections** are commonly transmitted by asymptomatic carriers at child care centers. Foul-smelling diarrhea usually is associated with abdominal distension and flatus. Diagnosis is confirmed by Giardia antigen in stool or three stools for ova and parasites.
   G. **Malabsorption** presents with chronic diarrhea, weight loss, poor appetite, weakness and decreased activity, bloating and flatulence, abdominal pain, and chronic vomiting. The most common causes are cystic fibrosis and celiac disease. Chronic diarrhea and failure to thrive warrants a sweat test. Screening for celiac disease consists of a D-xylose absorption test and a serum celiac disease panel (antigliadin, antiendomysial, and antireticulin antibodies). Celiac disease must be confirmed by intestinal biopsy.

IV. **Management of CNSD**
   A. Fluid intake should be reduced to less than 100 mL/kg/day. Water is substituted for juice to reduce the child's interest in drinking. Switching from the bottle to the cup also decreases fluid intake.
   B. Fat intake is increased to 4 g/kg/day by adding whole milk to the diet. If lactose

intolerance is present, low-lactose milk can be used or lactase drops can be added to milk. Butter, margarine, or vegetable oil are liberally added to foods for children less than 2 years of age.

C. Dietary fiber can be increased by consumption of fresh fruits and vegetables or by the addition of bran.

References, see page 164.

Constipation

Constipation is common in infants and children. The problem usually resolves after modification of the child's fluid and dietary regimen.

Pathophysiology

A. Persistent difficulty with the passage of stool may lead to impaction, stool withholding, and fecal soiling.

Conditions Associated With Constipation	
Condition	Common Causes
Lack of Fecal Bulk	High-carbohydrate or high-protein diet Undernutrition
Abnormally Hard Stools	Excessive cow milk intake
Abnormally Dry Stools	Dehydration Infantile renal acidosis Diabetes insipidus Idiopathic hypercalcemia
Nervous System Lesion	Spinal cord lesions
Mechanical Obstruction	Anorectal stenotic lesions Intrinsic and extrinsic masses Strictures Aganglionosis (Hirschsprung disease)
Diseases That Complicate Defecation	Amyotonia congenita Cerebral palsy Hypertonia Hypothyroidism

Neonates and infants younger than 1 year of age

A. Evaluation of constipation in neonates and infants

1. Inadequate fluid intake, undernutrition, and excessive cow milk intake should be excluded during the history.

2. Anal inspection at the time of birth reveals anorectal anomalies in one in every 2,500 live births. Anal stenosis accounts for 20% of these abnormalities. The anus appears very small with a central black dot of meconium, and the infant must make an intense effort to pass a ribbon-like stool. The abdomen may be distended and stool can often be palpated on abdominal examination.

3. Hirschsprung disease

a. Hirschsprung disease accounts for 20-25% of cases of neonatal obstructio and it is more common in males. Symptoms develop during the first mon of life in 80%. The majority of infants are unable to pass stool normally durir the first week.

b. Infants with Hirschsprung disease usually fail to pass meconium durir the first 48 hours of life. The abdomen is usually distended and tympaniti Abdominal peristaltic activity may be visible, and fecal masses may be palpabl The anal canal and rectum are empty of feces.

c. Plain abdominal radiographs reveal gas and stool in the colon above th rectum. A rectosigmoid index (the diameter of the rectum divided by th diameter of the sigmoid) of less than one is consistent with Hirschsprur disease.

d. When findings from the history, physical, and plain abdominal radiograph suggest Hirschsprung disease, contrast examination of the unprepare colon should be obtained. The diagnosis is confirmed by endoscopic biops

B. Management of simple constipation in infants

1. Dietary corrective measures are the initial therapy for infants with simple constipatio Increasing fluid intake and adding carbohydrate sugar to the formula ofte corrects the problem.

2. Infants that do not respond to dietary measures are treated with a minera oil preparation. Routine suppository administration, enemas, and stimula laxatives should be avoided.

III. Older infants and children

A. Evaluation

1. Fluid and dietary fiber intake should be assessed. Older children with chron constipation and stool withholding usually also have fecal incontinence.

2. Moveable fecal masses are often appreciated in the left colon and sigmoi

3. The lower back should be examined for a deep pilonidal dimple with hair tu and/or sacral agenesis, suggestive of myelodysplasia. Anal inspection ma reveal primary anal disease. Normal anal tone found on rectal examinatio indicates normal anal innervation. The rectal vault may be filled with inspissate stool.

4. Anteroposterior and lateral x-rays of the abdomen usually reveal a large rectal/rectosigmo impaction with variable amounts of stool throughout the remainder of the colo

B. Management of chronic constipation

1. **Distal impaction** should be removed with hypertonic phosphate enemas (Flee enema). Usually three enemas are administered during a 36- to 48-hour perio

2. **Mineral oil** should be prescribed. The initial dose of mineral oil is 30-75 m twice daily. Mineral oil is tasteless, and it can be taken with fruit juice, Kool-Ai or a soft drink. After one month, the oil is tapered by 15 mL (0.5 oz) per dose Haley's MO is a mineral oil solution of 1.4 gm/5 mL.

3. The child should sit on the toilet, with proper foot support, for five minutes afte the evening meal to take advantage of the gastrocolic reflex. A bulk-type stoo softener (eg, Metamucil) should be initiated when the mineral oil dosage ha been tapered to 15 mL twice daily.

References, see page 164.

Gastroenteritis

Acute gastroenteritis consists of diarrheal disease of rapid onset, often with nausea, vomiting, fever, or abdominal pain. It occurs an average of 1.3-2.3 times per year between the ages of 0 and 5 years. Most episodes of acute gastroenteritis will resolve within 3 to 7 days.

I. **Pathophysiology.** Gastroenteritis in children is caused by viral, bacterial, and parasitic organisms, although the vast majority of cases are viral or bacterial in origin.

II. **Viral gastroenteritis**
   A. All of the viruses produce watery diarrhea often accompanied by vomiting and fever, but usually not associated with blood or leukocytes in the stool or with prominent cramping.
   B. **Rotavirus** is the predominant viral cause of dehydrating diarrhea. Rotaviral infections tend to produce severe diarrhea, causing up to 70% of episodes in children under 2 years of age who require hospitalization. Rotavirus infection tends to occur in the fall in the southwest of the US, then sweeping progressively eastward, reaching the northeast by late winter and spring.
   C. **Norwalk viruses** are the major cause of large epidemics of acute nonbacterial gastroenteritis, occurring in schools, camps, nursing homes, cruise ships, and restaurants. **Enteric adenovirus** is the third most common organism isolated in infantile diarrhea.

III. **Bacterial gastroenteritis**
   A. The bacterial diarrheas are caused by elaboration of toxin (enterotoxigenic pathogens) or by invasion and inflammation of the mucosa (invasive pathogens).
   B. **Secretory diarrheas** are modulated through an enterotoxin, and the patient does not have fever or myalgias or tenesmus, or white or red blood cells in the stool. The diarrhea is watery, often is large in volume, and often associated with nausea and vomiting.
   C. **Invasive diarrhea** is caused by bacterial enteropathogens, and is accompanied by systemic signs, such as fever, myalgias, arthralgias, irritability, and loss of appetite. Cramps and abdominal pain are prominent. The diarrhea consists of frequent passing of small amounts of stool within the mucus. Stool examination reveals leukocytes, red blood cells, and often gross blood.

Acute Diarrhea Patterns and Associated Pathogens	
Secretory/enterotoxigenic	**Inflammatory**
Characterized by watery diarrhea and absence of fecal leukocytes	Characterized by dysentery (ie, fever and bloody stools), fecal leukocytes, and erythrocytes
Food poisoning (toxigenic)	
Staphylococcus aureus *Bacillus cereus* *Clostridium perfringens*	*Shigella* Invasive *E coli* *Salmonella* *Campylobacter*

Secretory/enterotoxigenic	Inflammatory
Enterotoxigenic	
Escherichia coli Vibrio cholera Giardia lamblia Cryptosporidium Rotavirus Norwalk-like virus	C difficile Entameba histolytica

IV. **General approach to the patient with gastroenteritis**
   A. **Determining and managing the fluid losses, dehydration and electrolyte abnormalities** is more important than ascertaining the specific microbiologic cause.
   B. **History** should assess recent antibiotic use, underlying diseases, other illnesses in the family, travel, untreated water, raw shellfish, attendance at a child care center, and foods eaten recently.

Clinical Evaluation and Treatment of Acute Diarrhea

Step One--Assess child for degree of dehydration

No dehydration	Continue oral hydration and feeding
Mild/severe dehydration--------->	Initiate rehydration by oral route (intravenous for severely dehydrated patients)

Step Two--Assess Clinical History for Etiologic Clues

Etiologic Clue	Etiology Suggested
Fever, crampy abdominal pain, tenesmus	Inflammatory colitis or ileitis
History of bloody stool	Shigella, enteroinvasive E coli, amebiasis, other bacterial causes
Fever and abdominal pain	Yersinia enterocolitis
Current or previous antibiotic use	Antibiotic-associated enteritis or pseudomemb-ranous colitis
Multiple cases and common food source	Incubation <6 hours: Staphylococcus aureus, Bacillus cereus Incubation >6 hours: Clostridium perfringens
Ingestion of inadequately cooked seafood	Vibrio parahaemolyticus
Recent measles, severe malnutrition, AIDS, other causes of immunosuppression	Bacterial (Salmonella), viral (rotavirus), or parasitic (isosporiasis, Cryptosporidium)

Step Three--Examine Stool:

	Indicated for:	Finding:	Etiology Suggested:
Visual examination	All patients	Gross blood	Dysentery, colitis, invasive organism
Microscopic examination for white/red blood cells	Patients who have had diarrhea >3 days, fever, blood in stool, weight loss	Red cells and leukocytes Red cells without leukocytes	Shigella, enterohemorrhagic EC, enteroinvasive EC, Campylobacter, Clostridium, E histolytica
Parasitic examination (wet mount, acid-fast staining, or concentration)	Diarrhea >10 days	Positive	Giardia, Amoeba, Cryptosporidium, Isospora, Strongyloides
Clostridium difficile toxin	Patients taking antibiotics	Positive	C difficile colitis

Assessment of Diarrheal Dehydration						
Clinical Finding	Mild (10-40 mL/kg)	Moderate (50-90 mL/kg)			Severe (100-130 mL/kg)	
Affect/sensorium	Normal	Irritability		Lethargy	Stupor	
Eyes	Normal		Sunken		Deeply sunken	
Mucous membrane	Normal		Dry		Very dry	
Tears when crying	Yes		No		No	
Thirst	Normal	+	++	+++	++++ or unresponsive	
Skin turgor (capillary refill)	Normal		Reduced (<1 sec)		Very reduced (2-3 sec)	
Fontanelle	Normal		Depressed		Severely depressed	
Pulse	Full	Full		Weak	Feeble or absent	
Pulse rate	Normal		Elevated		Very rapid	
Blood pressure	Normal		Normal		Low or absent	

C. Fluid therapy
   1. Mild-to-moderate dehydration
      a. **Mildly or moderately dehydrated children** should receive oral rehydration therapy (ORT) at 50 mL/kg (mild dehydration) or 100 mL/kg (moderate dehydration) over a 4-hour period. Replacement of stool losses (at 10 mL/kg for each stool) and of emesis (estimated volume) will require adding appropriate amounts of solution to the total.
      b. Use of cola, fruit juice and sports beverages are not recommended; their electrolyte content is inappropriate, and they contain too much carbohydrate.

2. **Prevention of dehydration.** Children who have diarrhea, but not dehydrated may be given glucose-electrolyte solution in addition to their regular diets to replace stool losses. The well-hydrated child should continue to consume an age-appropriate diet and drink more than the usual amounts of the normal fluids.

3. **Severely dehydrated children** who are in a state of shock must receive immediate and aggressive intravenous (IV) therapy. When the patient is stable, hydration may be continued orally.

4. **Intravenous rehydration**

   a. When intravenous rehydration is required, it should begin with an isotonic solution (normal saline, lactated Ringer). Severe dehydration clinically is associated with a loss of 10-12% of body weight in fluids and electrolytes (100 to 120 mL/kg); therefore, this amount plus additional losses should be infused.

   b. Infusion rates of up to 100 mL/min are appropriate in older children. Infusion rates of 40 mL/kg are given over the first 30 minutes, with the remainder of the deficit (70 mL/kg) over the next 2.5 hours, until the calculated fluid loss has been replenished.

   c. For infants, correction should be slower, with infusion rates no more than 30 mL/kg over the first hour and the remaining 70 mL/kg over 5 hours.

   d. Subsequent maintenance fluids should be given orally. Oral fluids should be initiated as soon as the patient can drink. They should be given simultaneously with intravenous fluids until the total fluids administered have replenished the calculated deficit.

D. **Antibiotic therapy.** The effectiveness of antimicrobial therapy is well established in shigellosis. Shigella is the cause of bacterial dysentery and is the second most commonly identified bacterial pathogen in diarrhea between the ages of 6 months and 10 years. It causes watery diarrhea with mucus and gross blood. Treatment consists of ceftriaxone or cefixime.

E. **Refeeding**

1. Children who have diarrhea and are not dehydrated should continue to be fed age-appropriate diets. Fatty foods and foods high in simple sugars, such as juices and soft drinks should be avoided. Well-tolerated foods include complex carbohydrates (rice, wheat, potatoes, bread, cereals), lean meats, yogurt, fruits, and vegetables. The BRAT diet (bananas, rice, applesauce, toast) does not supply optimal nutrition.

2. Introducing the child's regular form of milk early in the course of therapy is recommended.

F. **Antidiarrheal compounds** (eg, loperamide, diphenoxylate, bismuth compounds, Kaopectate) should not be used to treat acute diarrhea.

V. **Laboratory examinations**

A. The presence of blood in the stool, fever, or persistence of the diarrhea for more than 3 days may trigger a laboratory pursuit of an etiologic agent.

B. **Microscopic stool examination.** If erythrocytes and white blood cells are present, particularly in the setting of fever, a bacterial pathogen (Campylobacter, Yersinia, Salmonella, Shigella) should be suspected. Many red blood cells in the absence of white blood cells suggests the presence of Entamoeba.

C. **Stool culture** should be reserved for individuals whose diarrhea has not responded to fluid and feeding and for those who have fever and the presence of leukocytes or red blood cells in the stool.

References, see page 164.

Gastroesophageal Reflux

Gastroesophageal reflux (GER) is a common condition involving regurgitation. GER implies a functional or physiologic process in a healthy infant with no underlying systemic abnormalities. The prevalence of GER peaks between one to four months of age, and usually resolves by six to 12 months of age. Regurgitation occurs in 40 to 65 percent of healthy infants.

Gastroesophageal reflux disease (GERD) is a pathologic process in infants manifested by poor weight gain, signs of esophagitis, persistent respiratory symptoms, and changes in neurobehavior. GERD occurs in approximately one in 300 infants.

I. Clinical manifestations
   A. **Infants** with GER regurgitate without inadequate growth, esophagitis, or respiratory disease. Infants with GER are thriving and represent the majority of infants who present with this condition.
   B. Patients with GERD may manifest persistent regurgitation with secondary poor weight gain and failure to thrive. Other infants may manifest signs of esophagitis, including persistent irritability, pain, feeding problems, and iron deficiency anemia.

II. **Diagnostic evaluation.** In most cases of GER, no diagnostic study is required. Although scintigraphy may best quantify gastric emptying or aspiration, it is not as commonly used as the upper GI examination (barium fluoroscopy).

III. **Management**
   A. **Conservative treatment of GER** involves thickened feedings and positional changes in infants, and dietary modification in children. Healthy infants who regurgitate may be managed by thickening feedings with up to one tablespoon of dry rice cereal per 1 oz of formula.
   B. Smaller, more frequent feedings are recommended in older infants and children. Completely upright and prone positioning is beneficial in infants with GERD. Soft bedding materials should be avoided in this setting. Prone positioning is not routinely recommended as first-line management of simple regurgitation without evidence of GERD.
   C. **Pharmacologic management**
      1. *H_2-receptor antagonists*
         a. **Cimetidine (Tagamet).** The recommended starting dosage is 10 mg per kg per dose four times daily before meals and at bedtime for eight weeks. Potential side effects include headaches, dizziness, diarrhea, and gynecomastia.
         b. **Ranitidine (Zantac)** 1-2 mg per kg per dose two to three times daily (2-6 mg per kg per day) is the starting dosage. Potential side effects include headaches and malaise, but ranitidine has fewer central nervous system and anti-androgenic side effects.

Dosages and Side Effects of H_2-Receptor Agonists and Prokinetic Agents		
Agents	**Dosage**	**Side effects**
Cimetidine (Tagamet)	10 mg per kg per dose, four times daily	Headaches, dizziness, diarrhea, gynecomastia
Ranitidine (Zantac)	1 to 2 mg per kg per dose, two to three times daily	Headaches and malaise

Agents	Dosage	Side effects
Cisapride (Propulsid)*	0.2 mg per kg per dose, three to four times daily	Cardiac arrhythmia, diarrhea

*Because of the small potential risk of serious arrhythmias, this drug is only available via a limited access program.

2. **Prokinetic agent:** Cisapride (Propulsid) is the prokinetic of choice for GERD. It increases lower esophageal sphincter pressure and esophageal contractile amplitude. Reports of fatal arrhythmias have emerged. Cisapride is available through a limited access program if other therapies are not effective.

References, see page 164.

Inflammatory Bowel Disease

I. **Initial evaluation of chronic diarrhea**
 A. The initial diagnostic evaluation of chronic diarrhea includes stool cultures for enteric pathogens, tests for ova and parasites, Clostridium difficile toxin, and fecal leukocytes. Specific cultures for Yersinia enterocolitica, isolation of toxigenic strains of Escherichia coli, and serologic titers for Entamoeba histolytica may also be necessary.
 B. **Laboratory studies** include levels of C-reactive protein, which correlates with severity of disease, and levels of serum proteins (eg, albumin, transferrin, prealbumin, retinol-binding protein), which assess nutritional status. The degree of anemia indicates the severity of mucosal injury and duration of illness.
 C. **Colonoscopy or flexible sigmoidoscopy** with biopsy is valuable in characterizing mucosal injury.
 D. **Abdominal plain films** with the patient in upright and supine positions should be obtained in patients with severe disease to detect perforation, toxic megacolon, or thumbprinting.

II. **Ulcerative colitis**
 A. Ulcerative colitis (UC) is the most common cause of chronic colitis. Inflammation is localized primarily in the mucosa. The most common symptoms are abdominal pain, rectal bleeding, diarrhea, fever, and malaise.
 B. The incidence ranges from 4 to 15 cases per 100,000. Disease may present at any time but does so most often during adolescence and young adulthood, with a higher risk of the disease in young females than males. Among family members, the risk is tenfold higher. Ashkenazi Jews are afflicted more often than non-Jewish populations.
 C. Thirty percent of UC patients present with disease limited to the rectum, 40% have more extensive disease but not extending beyond the hepatic flexure, and 30% have total colonic involvement.
 D. **Diagnostic evaluation**
  1. Inflammation characteristically begins in the rectum. The mucosa is erythematous, friable, and edematous, with superficial erosions and ulcerations. Histologic features of ulcerative colitis include diffuse shallow ulceration of the mucosa, crypt abscesses, thickening of the muscularis mucosa, and pronounced inflammatory cell infiltration.
  2. **Extraintestinal manifestations**
   a. **Musculoskeletal.** Arthritis is the most common extraintestinal manifestation of ulcerative colitis. It is migratory, often involving the hip, ankle, wrist, or

elbow. It is usually monoarticular and asymmetric, and its course parallels that of the colitis. Ankylosing spondylitis and sacroiliitis, or axial arthritis, typically present as low back pain with morning stiffness.

b. **Ocular.** Episcleritis, uveitis, and iritis may occur.

c. **Dermatologic.** Abnormalities may include erythema nodosum, pyoderma gangrenosum, lichen planus, and aphthous ulcers.

d. **Hepatobiliary.** Manifestations may include hepatic steatosis, primary sclerosing cholangitis (4%), cholelithiasis, and pericholangitis.

e. **Miscellaneous.** Other complications include nephrolithiasis and a hypercoagulable state.

III. Crohn disease

A. Crohn disease (CD) is a chronic inflammatory process, which may involve any portion of the gastrointestinal tract from the mouth to the anus. Inflammation is characterized by transmural extension and irregular involvement of the intestinal tract, with intervening normal tissue ("skip areas"). Most often, the distal ileum and proximal colon are involved; in about 25% of cases, only the colon is affected.

B. Crohn disease often has its onset during adolescence and young adulthood. It is more common in females. The overall risk is two to four times higher in first-degree relatives.

C. Fever, abdominal pain, diarrhea, weight loss, and fatigue are common. Rectal bleeding is not as prominent a feature in Crohn disease as it is in ulcerative colitis. About 20% of patients have evidence of perianal disease, such as perirectal fistulas, anal skin tags, anal ulcerations or fissures, or perirectal abscesses. Crohn disease causes extra-intestinal manifestations like those of ulcerative colitis.

D. **Diagnostic evaluation**

1. Anemia, caused by chronic blood loss and a mildly elevated white blood cell count are common.

2. Endoscopic findings include focal ulcerations and inflammation is interrupted by skip areas. Other features of Crohn disease include rectal sparing, cobblestone appearance, strictures, and ileal involvement.

IV. Management of ulcerative colitis

A. **Mild-to-moderate cases of ulcerative colitis**

1. **Mesalamine (Asacol)** is an oral 5-ASA compound used for active ulcerative colitis, and olsalazine sodium (Dipentum) is used for maintenance therapy. The target dosage for the tablet Asacol (in divided doses) is 2.4 g/day, the capsule (Pentasa) 4 g/day, and capsule olsalazine (Dipentum) 1 g/day.

2. Limited left-sided colonic disease or rectosigmoid disease may respond to local therapy (enemas, suppositories) with corticosteroids and mesalamine.

3. Rectal preparations of mesalamine (Rowasa enema and suppository) can deliver higher concentrations to the distal colon for proctitis. Rowasa (4 g) is the only enema preparation of 5-ASA.

4. **Balsalazide (Colazal).** Balsalazide, a prodrug of mesalamine (5-aminosalicylic acid) for oral treatment of mildly to moderately active ulcerative colitis. Patients treated with balsalazide are more likely to achieve a symptomatic remission (88% vs 57%) or a complete remission (62% vs 37%), and became asymptomatic in 10 days compared to 25 days with delayed-release mesalamine.

B. **Moderately severe cases of ulcerative colitis**

1. These patients may require rehydration or blood transfusion. Corticosteroids, a low-residue diet, and local therapy should be initiated.

2. Prednisone usually is started at a dose of 1 to 2 mg/kg per day for 1 to 2 weeks. Once the patient is stabilized, the patient is weaned off the steroids to alternate-day therapy over 4 to 8 weeks; mesalamine (Asacol) is usually started. Hydrocortisone retention enema (Cortenema), is effective for distal ulcerative colitis.

C. Fulminant ulcerative colitis requires immediate hospitalization.
1. Fluid and electrolyte status must be stabilized and blood transfusions given as needed. Intravenous corticosteroids (methylprednisolone), broad-spectrum antibiotics (metronidazole, an aminoglycoside, and ampicillin), parenteral nutrition, and bowel rest are initiated.
2. If the patient deteriorates clinically or develops complications (hemorrhage, toxic megacolon), emergency surgery is performed. If the patient has not improved for 2 to 4 weeks after maximal medical therapy, a colectomy should be considered. Surgery is curative for UC.

Treatment of Inflammatory Bowel Disease

	Dose/day	Route	Side Effects
5-Aminosalicylic Acid			
Mesalamine (Asacol)	30-50 mg/kg	PO	Nephrotoxicity
Mesalamine (Rowasa)	2-4 g qd		Chills, diarrhea
Enema	500 mg bid	PR	
Suppository		PR	
Mesalamine (Pentasa)	50-60 mg/kg	PO	Local irritation
Olsalazine (Dipentum)	20-30 mg/kg	PO	Nephrotoxicity
Basalazine (Colazal)	2.25 g tid	PO	Watery diarrhea
Steroids			
Prednisone	1-2 mg/kg	PO	Osteoporosis, hypertension, poor growth, obesity, hirsutism, cataracts, adrenal suppression
Methylprednisolone	0.8-1.6 mg/kg	PO	Same as for prednisone
Hydrocortisone			
Enema	100 mg QD-BID	PR	Local irritation
Foam	80 mg QD-BID	PR	Same as enema
Immunosuppressants			
6-mercaptopurine	1-1.5 mg/kg	PO	Pancreatitis, bone marrow suppression
Azathioprine	1.5-2 mg/kg	PO	Same as for 6-mercaptopurine
Cyclosporine	2-4 mg/kg	IV	Nephrotoxicity
	4-6 mg/kg	PO	Hirsutism, hypertension
Antibiotics			
Metronidazole	10-20 mg/kg	PO/IV	Peripheral neuropathy, metallic taste

	Dose/day	Route	Side Effects
Miscellaneous			
Folic acid	1 mg	PO	

V. Management of Crohn disease. Treatment is similar to that of ulcerative colitis. Corticosteroids and mesalamine (Asacol) are the mainstays of therapy. Patients with severe colitis, massive weight loss, and significant systemic symptoms may need to be hospitalized. Prednisone can induce a remission in 70% of patients who have small bowel disease.

   A. **Antibiotics** (metronidazole and ciprofloxacin) are useful in mild-to-moderate CD and perianal disease.

   B. **Immunosuppressive agents.** Mercaptopurine and azathioprine are reserved for patients with continuous disease activity despite corticosteroid therapy. Cyclosporine may be beneficial in refractory patients.

   C. **Surgery** for Crohn disease is not curative. Indications include obstruction or intractable symptoms. Disease almost always recurs after surgery.

References, see page 164.

Persistent Vomiting

Vomiting is defined as the forceful expulsion of gastric contents through the mouth. Vomiting can be caused by a benign, self-limited process or it may be indicative of a serious underlying disorder.

I. Pathophysiology of vomiting

   A. Vomiting is usually preceded by nausea, increased salivation, and retching. It is distinct from regurgitation, which is characterized by passive movement of gastric contents into the esophagus.

   B. Projectile vomiting results from intense gastric peristaltic waves, usually secondary to gastric outlet obstruction caused by hypertrophic pyloric stenosis or pylorospasm.

   C. Retching often precedes vomiting and is characterized by spasmodic contraction of the expiratory muscles with simultaneous abdominal contraction.

II. Clinical evaluation of vomiting

Etiology of Vomiting by Age			
	Newborn	**Infant**	**Older Child**
Obstruction	Malrotation of bowel Volvulus Intestinal atresia Intestinal stenosis Meconium ileus Meconium plug Hirschsprung disease Imperforate anus Incarcerated hernia	Pyloric stenosis Foreign bodies Malrotation (volvulus) Duplication of alimentary tract Intussusception Meckel diverticulum Hirschsprung disease Incarcerated hernia	Intussusception Foreign bodies Malrotation (volvulus) Meckel diverticulum Hirschsprung disease Incarcerated hernia Adhesions

	Newborn	Infant	Older Child
Gastrointestinal disorders (infectious/inflammatory)	Necrotizing enterocolitis Gastroesophageal reflux Paralytic ileus Peritonitis Milk allergy	Gastroenteritis Gastroesophageal reflux Pancreatitis Appendicitis Celiac disease Paralytic ileus Peritonitis	Gastroenteritis Peptic ulcer disease
Infectious disorders (nongastrointestinal)	Sepsis Meningitis	Sepsis Meningitis Otitis media Pneumonia Pertussis Hepatitis Urinary tract infection	Meningitis Otitis media Pharyngitis Pneumonia Hepatitis Urinary tract infection
Neurologic disorders	Hydrocephalus Kernicterus Subdural hematoma Cerebral edema	Hydrocephalus Subdural hematoma Intracranial hemorrhage Mass lesion (abscess, tumor)	Subdural hematoma Intracranial hemorrhage Brain tumor Other mass-occupying lesion Migraine Motion sickness Hypertensive encephalopathy
Metabolic and endocrine disorders	Inborn errors of metabolism: Urea cycle defects, galactosemia, disorders of organic acid metabolism Congenital adrenal hyperplasia Neonatal tetany	Inborn errors of metabolism Fructose intolerance Adrenal insufficiency Metabolic acidosis	Adrenal insufficiency Diabetic ketoacidosis
Renal disorders	Obstructive uropathy Renal insufficiency	Obstructive uropathy Renal insufficiency	Obstructive uropathy Renal insufficiency
Toxins		Digoxin Iron	Digoxin Iron Lead Food poisoning
Other			Pregnancy Anorexia nervosa Bulimia Psychogenic etiology

A. **Clinical evaluation of vomiting in the neonate**
1. **Bilious vomiting**, at any age, suggests intestinal obstruction or systemic infection. Anatomic abnormalities of the gastrointestinal tract that may present in the first week of life with bilious vomiting and abdominal distention include malrotation, volvulus, duplications of the bowel, bowel atresia, meconium plug, meconium ileus, incarcerated hernia, and aganglionosis (Hirschsprung disease).

2. **Necrotizing enterocolitis**
   a. NEC is the most common inflammatory condition of the intestinal tract in the neonate. Symptoms of NEC include abdominal distention, bilious vomiting, and blood in the stool.
   b. The infant who has NEC also may present with nonspecific signs of systemic infection, such as lethargy, apnea, temperature instability, and shock. NEC occurs mainly in preterm infants, although 10% of affected newborns present at term.

3. **Metabolic disorders**
   a. **Inborn errors of metabolism** should be considered in any acute neonatal illness, including persistent vomiting. Factors that suggest a metabolic disorder include early or unexplained death of a sibling, multiple spontaneous maternal abortions, or history of consanguinity.
   b. Associated features may include lethargy, hypotonia, and convulsions.

4. **Neurologic disorders.** Central nervous system abnormalities, such as intracranial hemorrhage, hydrocephalus and cerebral edema, should be suspected in the neonate who has neurologic deficits, a rapid increase in head circumference, or an unexplained fall in hematocrit.

B. **Clinical evaluation of vomiting in infancy**
   1. **Pyloric stenosis**
      a. Pyloric stenosis is a major consideration in infants. Hypertrophy of the pylorus causes gastric outlet obstruction at the pyloric canal. Five percent of infants whose parents had pyloric stenosis develop this disorder. Males are affected more often than females.
      b. Symptoms of pyloric stenosis usually begin at age 2 to 3 weeks, but may occur at birth or present as late as 5 months. An olive-size mass may be palpable in the right upper quadrant.

   2. **Gastroesophageal reflux**
      a. Gastroesophageal reflux (GER) is defined as retrograde movement of gastric contents into the esophagus. GER occurs in 65% of infants and is caused by inappropriate relaxation of the lower esophageal sphincter.
      b. GER is considered "pathologic" if symptoms persist beyond 18 to 24 months and/or if significant complications develop, such as failure to thrive, recurrent episodes of bronchospasm and pneumonia, apnea, or reflux esophagitis.

   3. **Gastrointestinal allergy.** Cow milk allergy is rare in infancy and early childhood and generally resolves by 2 to 3 years of age. Vomiting, diarrhea, colic and gastrointestinal loss of blood may occur.

II. **Clinical evaluation of vomiting in childhood**
A. **Peptic ulcer** in early childhood is often associated with vomiting. Peptic ulcer disease should be suspected if there is a family history of ulcer disease, or if there is hematemesis or unexplained iron deficiency anemia. Abdominal pain typically wakes the patient from sleep.

B. **Pancreatitis**
   1. Pancreatitis is a relatively rare cause of vomiting, but should be considered in the child who has sustained abdominal trauma. Patients usually complain of epigastric pain, which may radiate to the mid-back.
   2. Other factors predisposing to pancreatitis include viral illnesses (mumps), drugs (steroids, azathioprine), congenital anomalies of the biliary or pancreatic ducts, cholelithiasis, hypertriglyceridemia, and a family history of pancreatitis.

C. **Central nervous system disorders.** Persistent vomiting without other gastrointestinal or systemic complaints suggests an intracranial tumor or increased intracranial pressure. Subtle neurologic findings (eg, ataxia, head tilt) should be assessed and a detailed neurologic examination should be performed.

IV. **Physical examination of the child with persistent vomiting**
   A. **Volume depletion** often results from vomiting, manifesting as sunken fontanelles, decreased skin turgor, dry mouth, absence of tears, and decreased urine output.
   B. **Peritoneal irritation** should be suspected when the child keeps his knees drawn up or bends over. Abdominal distension, visible peristalsis, and increased bowel sounds suggests intestinal obstruction.
   C. **Abnormal masses, enlarged organs, guarding or tenderness** should be sought. A hypertrophic pylorus may manifest as a palpable "olive" in the right upper quadrant.
   D. **Intussusception** is often associated with a tender, sausage-shaped mass in the right upper quadrant and an empty right lower quadrant (Dance sign).
   E. **Digital rectal exam.** Decreased anal sphincter tone and large amounts of hard fecal material in the ampulla suggests fecal impaction. Constipation, increased rectal sphincter tone, and an empty rectal ampulla suggests Hirschsprung disease.

V. **Laboratory evaluation**
   A. **Serum electrolytes should be obtained** when dehydration is suspected.
   B. **Urinalysis** may detect a urinary tract infection or suggest the presence of a metabolic disorder.
   C. **Plasma amino acids and urine organic acids** should be measured if metabolic disease is suspected because of recurrent, unexplained episodes of metabolic acidosis.
   D. **Serum ammonia should be obtained in cases of cyclic vomiting** to exclude a urea cycle defect.
   E. **Liver chemistries and serum ammonia and glucose levels** should be obtained if liver disease is suspected.
   F. **Serum amylase** is frequently elevated in patients who have acute pancreatitis. Serum lipase levels may be more helpful because it remains elevated for a number of days following an acute episode.

VI. **Imaging studies**
   A. **Ultrasonography** of the abdomen is the initial imaging test for suspected pyloric stenosis; however, two-thirds of vomiting infants will have a negative sonogram and will subsequently require an upper gastrointestinal series.
   B. **Plain radiographs of the abdomen**
      1. **Supine and upright or left lateral decubitus radiographic views** are necessary for detecting congenital anatomic malformations or obstructive lesions.
      2. **Air-fluid levels** suggest obstruction, although this finding is nonspecific and may be seen with gastroenteritis.
      3. **Free air** in the abdominal cavity indicates a perforated viscus. Upright plain films may demonstrate free air under the diaphragm.
   C. **Upper gastrointestinal series** with nonionic, iso-osmolar, water-soluble contrast is indicated when anatomic abnormalities and/or conditions that cause gastric outlet obstruction are suspected.
   D. **Barium enema** should be performed to detect lower intestinal obstruction, and it may also be therapeutic in intussusception.

VII. **Treatment**
   A. **Initial therapy** should correct hypovolemia and electrolyte abnormalities. In acute diarrheal illnesses with vomiting, oral rehydration therapy is usually adequate for treatment of dehydration.
   B. **Bilious vomiting and suspected intestinal obstruction** is managing by giving nothing by mouth, and by placing a nasogastric tube connected to intermittent suction. Bilious vomiting requires surgical consultation.

C. Pharmacologic therapy

1. **Antiemetic agents** usually are not required because most instances of acute vomiting are caused by self-limited, infectious gastrointestinal illnesses. Antiemetic drugs may be indicated for postoperative emesis, motion sickness, cytotoxic drug-evoked emesis, and gastroesophageal reflux disease.

2. **Diphenhydramine and dimenhydrinate** are useful in treating the symptoms of motion sickness or vestibulitis.

3. **Prochlorperazine and chlorpromazine** have anticholinergic and antihistaminic properties and are used to treat vomiting caused by drugs, radiation, and gastroenteritis.

References, see page 164.

Neurologic and Rheumatic Disorders

Febrile Seizures

Febrile seizures are the most common convulsive disorder of childhood. A febrile seizur is defined as a seizure associated with fever in infancy or early childhood (usually betwee 3 months and 5 years of age) without evidence of intracranial infection or other cause

The problem almost always resolves without sequelae. Only a small minority w develop non-febrile seizures later. There is no risk of brain damage.

I. **Epidemiology.** Febrile seizures occur in 2-4% of young children. The most commo age of onset is in the second year of life. Higher temperature and a history of febril seizures in a close relative are risk factors for the development of a febrile seizure

A. **Recurrence**
   1. After the first febrile seizure, 33% of children will experience one or more febril seizures, and 9% of children who have febrile seizures will have 3 or more The younger the child's age when the first febrile seizure occurs, the greate the likelihood of recurrence.
   2. Family history of febrile seizures is a risk factor for recurrence. Short duratio of fever before the initial seizure and relatively lower fever at the time of th initial seizure are risk factors.

B. **Epilepsy.** Fewer than 5% of children who have febrile seizures develop epilepsy Risk factors for the development of epilepsy following febrile seizures includ suspicious or abnormal development before the first seizure, family history c afebrile seizures, and complex first febrile seizure.

II. **Pathophysiology.** Most febrile illnesses associated with febrile seizures are cause by common infections (tonsillitis, upper respiratory infections, otitis media). Childre of preschool age are subject to frequent infections and high fevers.

III. **Clinical evaluation**

A. Febrile seizures usually occur early in the course of a febrile illness, often as th first sign. The seizure may be of any type, but the most common is tonic-clonic Initially there may be a cry, followed by loss of consciousness and muscular rigidity During this tonic phase, apnea and incontinence may occur. The tonic phas is followed by the clonic phase of repetitive, rhythmic jerking movements, whic is then followed by postictal lethargy or sleep.

B. Other seizure types may be characterized by staring with stiffness or limpness or only focal stiffness or jerking. Most seizures last less than 6 minutes; 8% las longer than 15 minutes.

C. An underlying illness that may require treatment should be sought. Symptom of infection, medication exposure, or trauma should be assessed. Family histor of febrile or afebrile seizures should be evaluated. A complete description of th seizure should be obtained from a witness.

D. **Physical examination**
   1. The level of consciousness, presence of meningismus, a tense or bulging fontanelle Kernig or Brudzinski sign, and any focal abnormalities in muscle strength o tone should be sought.
   2. Encephalitis or meningitis must be excluded.

E. **Laboratory studies** should evaluate the source of fever. A lumbar puncture (LP is indicated if there is any suspicion of meningitis. CT or MRI are seldom helpfu and are not performed routinely. The electroencephalogram (EEG) is not helpfu in the evaluation of febrile seizures because it is not predictive of recurrence risl of later epilepsy.

Ⅶ. Management of febrile seizures

A. The child should be kept in the emergency department or physician's office for at least several hours and re-evaluated. Most children will have improved and be alert, and the child may be sent home if the cause of the fever has been diagnosed and treated. Hospital admission is necessary if the child is unstable or if meningitis remains a possibility.

B. Parental counseling

1. Parents are advised that febrile seizures do not cause brain damage, and the likelihood of developing epilepsy or recurrent non-febrile seizures is very small. There is a risk of further febrile seizures during the current or subsequent febrile illnesses.

2. If another seizure occurs, the parent should place the child on his side or abdomen with the face downward. Nothing should be forced between the teeth. If the seizure does not stop after 10 minutes, the child should be brought to the hospital.

C. Control of fever with antipyretics (acetaminophen) and sponging is recommended, but this practice has not been proven to lower the risk of recurrent febrile seizures.

D. Childhood immunizations. Febrile seizures occur most commonly following a DPT immunization because pertussis provokes fever. The advantages of vaccines must be weighed against the risk of pertussis if immunization is postponed.

Ⅶ. Long-term management

A. Prophylaxis with diazepam or phenobarbital is not routinely necessary, but is reserved for very young children who have sustained multiple seizures associated with focal post-ictal paralysis.

B. Diazepam may be administered orally and rectally during febrile illnesses to prevent recurrences of seizures. Oral diazepam is given in three divided doses to a total of 1 mg/kg per day when the child is ill or feverish.

References, see page 164.

Seizures and Epilepsy

Approximately 1 to 2 percent of the U.S. population has epilepsy. The term "seizure" designates a clinical event that represents dysfunction of the central nervous system (CNS) and may signal a serious underlying abnormality; however, in children the seizures usually result from a transient disturbance of brain function.

Ⅰ. Epidemiology and classification of seizure types

A. The ages of greatest risk for nonfebrile seizures are during infancy, childhood, and adolescence. The annual incidence rate from birth to 20 years of age is 0.56 per 1000. The two primary forms of epilepsy are generalized seizures and partial seizures.

B. **Partial seizures** are the most common form of epilepsy in children.

1. **Simple partial seizures (SPS)**

a. During simple partial seizures the child remains conscious and is able to verbalize throughout the seizure. Most SPS are focal, asynchronous, clonic or tonic motor movements, such as forced deviation of the head and eyes to one side.

b. An SPS typically is short-lived, rarely persisting longer than 10 to 20 seconds. The EEG characteristics shows unilateral spikes or sharp waves in the anterior temporal region.

2. **Complex partial seizures (CPS)**

a. CPS initially may be similar in appearance to an SPS, but they are followed

by impairment of consciousness. CPS may begin with a loss of consciousnes
The average duration of a CPS is 1 to 2 minutes.

   b. **Aura** signals the onset of a seizure in 30% of children who have CPS, wi
   the child complaining of epigastric discomfort, fear, or an unpleasant feelin

   c. **Automatisms** are repetitive, stereotyped behaviors. These are the hallma
   of CPS and occur in 50-75%. Automatisms follow the loss of consciousnes
   but unlike aura, the child is not aware of their presence. Automatisms ma
   include lip smacking, chewing, repetitive swallowing, excessive salivatio
   picking and pulling at clothing, constant rubbing of objects, and walkin
   and running. Automatisms are often associated with a fearful expressio

   d. During the partial seizure, the epileptiform discharge may spread from th
   temporal lobe to throughout the cortex, causing a generalized tonic-clon
   convulsion (termed secondary generalization).

   e. During CPS, the EEG is characterized by sharp waves or spike discharge
   in the anterior temporal or frontal lobe, or by multifocal spikes.

International Classification of Epileptic Seizures

Partial Seizures
   –Simple partial (consciousness retained)
   –Complex partial (consciousness impaired)
   –Partial seizure with secondary generalization

Generalized Seizures
   –Absence seizures
   –Myoclonic seizures
   –Clonic seizures
   –Tonic seizures
   –Tonic-clonic seizures
   –Atonic seizures

Unclassified Seizures

   C. **Generalized seizures**

   1. **Simple absence seizures** usually have their onset at 5 to 6 years of ag
   and are characterized by brief (5-20 sec) lapses in consciousness, speecl
   or motor activity. Absence seizures are not accompanied by an aura or a postict
   drowsiness, but automatisms may occur (consisting of eye blinking or lip smacking
   The EEG is characterized by 3 per second generalized spike and wave discharge

   2. **Atypical absence** seizures are characterized by myoclonic movements
   the face and body. The EEG shows 2-2.5 per second or 3.5-4.5 per secon
   generalized spike and wave discharges.

   3. **Myoclonic seizures** are characterized by brief, often repetitive, symmetri
   muscle contractions with loss of body tone.

   4. **Atonic seizures** cause the child to fall because of a sudden loss of postura
   tone.

   5. **Tonic or clonic seizures** are characterized by a sudden loss of consciousnes
   and tonic-clonic, tonic, or clonic contractions. The child may develop perior
   cyanosis and loss of bladder control. The seizure is followed by a 30- to 60-minut
   period of deep sleep and postictal headache.

II. **Pathophysiology of epilepsy**

   A. The etiology of most seizures in children remains unknown.

   B. The acute onset of seizures may result from head injury, CNS infection (meningiti
   encephalitis), cerebrovascular diseases (infarction, arteriovenous malformatio

hemorrhage, venous thrombosis), toxins (lead), brain tumor, specific epilepsy syndromes, genetic/hereditary diseases (Down syndrome, tuberous sclerosis), metabolic and systemic diseases (endocrine, renal), degenerative disorders (leukodystrophy), or hereditary malformations.

C. **Hypoxic-ischemic encephalopathy** is the most common cause of seizures in the newborn. Children who have neonatal seizures following a hypoxic-ischemic insult are at significant risk to continue to have seizures.

D. **Pyridoxine dependency** may be the cause of seizures that begin shortly after birth.

E. **Metabolic encephalopathies** commonly are associated with seizures in the newborn. A urea cycle abnormality or a disorder of amino acid metabolism may cause seizures.

F. **Structural abnormalities of the brain and congenital disorders** of neuronal migration play an important role in the causation of epilepsy. Simple febrile seizures are not a cause of epilepsy.

I. Diagnosis

A. A presumptive diagnosis of epilepsy generally is made from a history of spontaneous recurrent seizures and physical examination findings. The parent usually can give a good account of the seizure and whether it was generalized or focal in onset. The child may reveal the existence of aura, which signifies a focal onset.

B. **Routine EEG** may be useful in supporting a clinical diagnosis of epilepsy by showing epileptiform discharges (eg, spikes or sharp waves). Routine EEG is not highly sensitive, and fewer than 50 percent of routine EEGs are abnormal in patients who are known to have epilepsy. Many patients with epilepsy have normal EEGs.

C. **EEG-video monitoring**. A definitive diagnosis of epilepsy can only be made using EEG-video monitoring. The correlation between clinical semiology and ictal EEG also allows epilepsy to be categorized as partial or generalized and for the zone of seizure onset to be located.

D. **Ambulatory EEG** allows the recording of electrographic seizures but does not permit correlation between EEG and seizure semiology. Ambulatory EEG can be a useful extension of routine EEG. It does not replace EEG-video monitoring.

E. **Invasive EEG** is necessary only when surgery is being considered and a regular EEG evaluation fails to identify the zone of seizure onset.

F. **MRI** is useful for excluding structural brain disorders.

G. **Fasting blood glucose and serum calcium levels** are indicated if the history suggests hypoglycemia or hypocalcemia as a cause of the seizure.

V. Management of nonfebrile seizures

A. **Anticonvulsant medication**

1. Anticonvulsants are initiated following absence seizures, myoclonic seizures, and infantile spasms because the risk of recurrence is high.

2. A single afebrile tonic-clonic seizure has a 75% probability of not recurring if the neurologic examination and EEG are normal and there is no family history of epilepsy. Anticonvulsants are not advised following the initial tonic-clonic seizure in these children.

3. When two or more unprovoked afebrile seizures occur within a 6- to 12-month period, anticonvulsants usually are indicated.

Common Anticonvulsant Drugs				
Drug	Seizure Type	Oral Dose	Serum Level mcg/mL	Side Effects and Toxicities
Carbamazepine (Tegretol), carbamazepine XR (Tegretol XR)	Partial epilepsy Tonic-clonic	Begin 10 mg/kg/d. Increase by 5 mg/kg/d every wk to 20-30 mg/kg/d in 2 or 3 divided doses	4-12	Dizziness, drowsiness, diplopia, liver, dysfunction, anemia, leukopenia
Clonazepam (Klonopin)	Myoclonic Absence	Begin 0.05 mg/kg/d. Increase by 0.05 mg/kg per wk. Maximum, 0.2 mg/kg/d in 2 or 3 divided doses	6.3-56.8	Drowsiness, irritability, drooling, behavioral abnormalities, depression
Ethosuximide (Zarontin)	Absence Myoclonic	Begin 10 to 20 mg/kg/d in 2 divided doses; may be increased to 50 mg/kg/d	40-160	Drowsiness, nausea, rarely blood dyscrasias
Felbamate (Felbatol)	Partial epilepsy Tonic-clonic	600 to 1,200 mg/ 2,400 to 3,600 mg two to three times daily		Headache, insomnia, aplastic anemia, hepatitis
Gabapentin (Neurontin)	Partial epilepsy Tonic-clonic	Begin 300 mg/d. Increase by 300 mg/d every 3 to 5 days. Maximum 900 to 1200 mg/d in 3 equally divided doses	<2	Somnolence, dizziness, ataxia, headache, tremor, vomiting, nystagmus, fatigue, weight gain
Lamotrigine (Lamictal)	Partial epilepsy Tonic-clonic Lennox-Gastaut	Begin 2 mg/kg/d in 2 equal doses. Increase to maintenance dose of 5 to 15 mg/kg/d.	1-4	Severe rashes, drowsiness, headache, blurred vision
Topiramate (Topamax)	Partial epilepsy Tonic-clonic	Begin 25 to 50 mg Increase to 200 to 400 mg/day in 2 doses		Nephrolithiasis, paresthesias, weight loss
Tiagabine (Gabitril)	Partial epilepsy	Begin 4 mg Increase to 32 to 64 mg in 2-4 doses		Narrow spectrum of activity
Oxcarbazepine (Trileptal)	Partial epilepsy	Begin 300 to 600 mg Increase to 600 to 2,400 mg in 2 doses		Hyponatremia

Drug	Seizure Type	Oral Dose	Serum Level mcg/mL	Side Effects and Toxicities
Levetiracetam (Keppra)	Focal epilepsy	Begin 1,000 mg Increase to 1,000 to 3,000 mg in 2 doses		
Zonisamide (Zonegran)	Focal epilepsy	Begin 100 to 200 mg Increase to 400 to 600 mg every day in 2 doses		Nephrolithiasis, weight loss
Phenobarbital	Tonic-clonic Partial epilepsy	3 to 5 mg/kg/d in 1 or 2 divided doses	15-40	Hyperactivity, irritability, short attention span, temper tantrums, altered sleep pattern, Stevens-Johnson syndrome, depression of cognitive function
Phenytoin (Dilantin)	Partial epilepsy Tonic-clonic	5 m 6 mg/kg/d in 2 divided doses	10-20	Hirsutism, gum hypertrophy, ataxia, skin rash, Stevens Johnson syndrome
Primidone (Mysoline)	Tonic-clonic Partial epilepsy Myoclonic	Begin 50 mg/d in two divided doses. Gradually increase to 150 to 500 mg/d divided into 3 equal doses.	5-12	Aggressive behavior and personality changes similar to those for pheno-barbital
Sodium valproate (Depakote)	Tonic-clonic Absence Myoclonic Partial epilepsy Unclassified	Begin 10 mg/kg/d. Increase by 5 to 10 mg/kg per wk. Usual dose, 20 to 60 mg/kg/d in 2 or 3 divided doses.	50-100	Weight gain, alopecia, tremor, hepatotoxicity
Vigabatrin (Sabril)	Partial epilepsy	Begin 30 to 40 mg/kg/d. Increase by 10 mg/kg per wk. Maximum, 80 to 100 mg/kg/d in 2 equal doses	1.4-14	Agitation, drowsiness, weight gain, dizziness, headache, ataxia

B. **Felbamate (Felbatol)** has a broad spectrum of activity in both partial and generalized seizures, but rare reports of fatal aplastic anemia and hepatic failure limit its use.

C. **Gabapentin (Neurontin)** has excellent tolerability. It is not protein bound, has no appreciable hepatic metabolism and is excreted by the kidneys. Thus, gabapentin is appropriate for use in patients who require relatively quick titration, who have multiple drug intolerances or who are taking multiple drugs with the potential for interaction.

D. **Lamotrigine (Lamictal)** has a broad spectrum of activity against multiple seizure types. Sedation is notably rare, and it has an "alerting" response in some patients. One side effect is a rash. In less than 1 percent, the rash may progress to Stevens-Johnson syndrome, which can be life-threatening.

E. **Topiramate (Topamax)** has a broad spectrum of activity. Weight loss has been noted, which can be a desirable lateral side effect. Nephrolithiasis is rare; paresthesias are common.

F. **Tiagabine (Gabitril)** has no significant adverse side effects, but it has a relatively narrow spectrum of activity and must be titrated slowly.

G. **Levetiracetam (Keppra)** is unique among the new antiepileptic drugs because it is effective starting with the initial dose. It also has a mechanism of action that appears to be different from that of other antiepileptic drugs, and its tolerability and pharmacokinetics are very attractive. Drug interactions are minimal.

H. **Zonisamide (Zonegran)** has been used in Japan for 11 years and benefits from a large patient exposure, which supports its safety. Nephrolithiasis and weight loss may occur.

I. **Fosphenytoin (Cerebyx)** is a reformulated version of phenytoin for use in the treatment of status epilepticus.

J. **Long-acting carbamazepine (Tegretol XR)** allows for a twice-daily dosing that was not possible with the earlier version of carbamazepine. Oxcarbazepine (Trileptal) is a better-tolerated reformulation of carbamazepine. Intravenous valproate sodium (Depacon) can be useful for replacement in an acute setting or for rapid loading.

K. **Rectal diazepam (Diastat)** can be self-administered by patients who have seizure clusters to abort impending status epilepticus.

L. **Midazolam (Versed) and propofol (Diprivan)** may soon become standard therapy for status epilepticus because of their very short half-life, which allows rapid titration based on the EEG.

M. **Ketogenic diet.** The ketogenic diet uses ketosis and acidosis. A high-fat low-carbohydrate diet induces a starvation-like ketosis and acidosis, which has anticonvulsant effects. The diet is initiated in the hospital with starvation until ketones are present in the urine. The diet is indicated for use primarily in young children with intractable symptomatic generalized epilepsy of the Lennox-Gastaut type. Overall, 30 to 50 percent of children respond favorably.

N. **Vagus nerve stimulation.** The mechanism of action of vagus nerve stimulation (VNS) is likely mediated by the widespread afferent connections of the vagus nerve. Efficacy is comparable to adjunctive antiepileptic drugs. Efficacy may increase over time. VNS has no significant toxicity. Trials for its use in the treatment of depression are ongoing.

O. **Epilepsy surgery.** Seizures are intractable in approximately 20 percent of patients with epilepsy. Surgery is now a well-accepted modality for the treatment of medically

intractable epilepsy.
References, see page 164.

Headache

Chronic or recurrent headaches occur 75% of children by 15 years.

I. Clinical evaluation

  A. Headaches are characterized as isolated acute, recurrent acute, chronic nonprogressive, or chronic progressive. A social and educational history may identify significant stresses. Analgesic use should be determined.

  B. Physical examination should include measurement of growth parameters, head circumference, and blood pressure. The teeth should be examined and sinusitis should be sought. An arteriovenous malformation may cause an asymmetric, machinery-like cranial bruit.

  C. Papilledema. The presence of retinal venous pulsation on funduscopy provides evidence of normal intracranial pressure. Visual acuity should be measured, and a detailed neurologic examination is essential.

  D. Investigations. If increased intracranial pressure or an intracranial lesion is suspected, a computed tomographic (CT) head scan should be performed. Magnetic resonance imaging (MRI) may be required to diagnose subtle vascular abnormalities or hypothalamopituitary lesions.

  E. Lumbar puncture may be helpful if pseudotumor cerebri is suspected. However, lumbar puncture may result in herniation of the brain in patients who have obstructive hydrocephalus, an intracranial mass lesion, or cerebral edema. Neuroimaging should be performed prior to the lumbar puncture.

Physical and Neurological Examination of the Child with Headaches	
Feature	**Significance**
Growth parameters	Chronic illness may affect linear growth Hypothalamopituitary dysfunction may disturb growth
Head circumference	Increased intracranial pressure prior to fusion of the sutures may accelerate head growth
Skin	Evidence of trauma or a neurocutaneous disorder
Blood pressure	Hypertension
Neurologic examination	Signs of increased intracranial pressure Neurologic abnormality
Cranial bruits	May reflect an intracranial arteriovenous malformation

- F. Migraine
  1. Migraines may be associated with a preceding aura, which usually involves visual phenomena. The headache is usually unilateral or bilateral, recurrent, throbbing, and associated with nausea or vomiting. Photophobia or phonophobia is common.
  2. A family history of migraine is obtained in up to 80% of children who have migraine. A family history of motion sickness is common. Migraine episodes may be triggered by stress, lack of sleep, excitement, menstruation, or certain foods.

- II. Migraine management
  - A. Management of acute episodes
    1. Oral promethazine (Phenergan), 1 mg/kg up to 25 mg, often results in sleep and is generally effective. Intramuscular chlorpromazine (Compazine), 1 mg/kg, can be used for severe attacks.
    2. Simple analgesics, such as acetaminophen, ibuprofen, or naproxen, may be effective.
    3. Sumatriptan (Imitrex), a selective 5-HT agonist, is an effective treatment for migraine. The subcutaneous dose of 6 mg is effective and safe in school-age children. Oral and intranasal sumatriptan spray are less effective.
    4. Intravenous dihydroergotamine mesylate (DHE) is often effective when used with metoclopramide. Metoclopramide can be given orally or intravenously prior to the DHE, which is administered over 3 minutes at a dose of 0.5 to 1 mg. The DHE can be repeated every 8 hours. A nasal spray formulation of DHE is effective.

Treatment of Acute Migraine Episodes	
Simple analgesics	
Acetaminophen	Initial dose of 20 mg/kg PO, followed by 10 to 15 mg/kg q 4 h up to a maximum dose of 65 mg/kg per day (maximum, 3,000 mg/day)
Ibuprofen (Advil)	*1 to 12 years:* 10 mg/kg PO q 4 to 6 h *More than 12 years:* 200 to 400 mg PO q 4 h; maximum dose 1,200 mg/day
Naproxen (Aleve)	5 mg/kg PO q 12 h; maximum dose 750 mg/day
Antiemetics	
Promethazine (Phenergan)	Initial dose of 1 mg/kg PO (maximum, 25 mg); can be repeated at doses of 0.25 to 1 mg/kg q 4 to 6 h
Chlorpromazine (Compazine)	1 mg/kg IM for severe attacks
Other Drugs	
Sumatriptan (Imitrex)	6 mg SC; may repeat in 1-2 hours; max 12 mg/day Oral: 25-50 mg PO once; may repeat in 2 hours Intranasal: 5, 10, or 20 mg in one nostril; may repeat after 2 hours
Dihydroergotamine (DHE)	0.5 to 1 mg IV over 3 min in children >10 y. Can be repeated q8h. Used with metoclopramide.

B. Migraine prophylaxis. Migraine may be precipitated by stress, certain foods, lack of sleep, hormonal changes during the menstrual cycle, alcohol, and oral contraceptives. Elimination of these factors may reduce the frequency of the attacks.

Prophylactic Agents for Migraine	
Amitriptyline (Elavil)	5-10 mg qhs
Propranolol (Inderal)	1 to 4 mg/kg per day; start at low dose and increase slowly

References, see page 164.

Kawasaki Syndrome

Kawasaki syndrome (KS) is an acute, febrile, self-limited, infectious, multisystem vasculitis, which occurs in young children. Fever is often prolonged, and coronary aneurysms may lead to myocardial infarction and death.

I. **Epidemiology**
   A. Kawasaki syndrome has a peak incidence between 1 and 2 years of age. The disease is rare in children older than 8 years old, and it is uncommon before 3 months of age.
   B. Boys are affected more often than girls by a ratio of 1.5 to 1. Japanese and Korean children are at greatest risk (145 per 100,000). The rate for European children is 9 per 100,000, and the rate for African children is 20 per 100,000.

II. **Pathophysiology**
   A. Kawasaki syndrome is a multisystem vasculitis with a predilection for the coronary arteries, associated with pancarditis and pericarditis. Death during this phase is usually caused by an arrhythmia, although fatal heart failure may sometimes occur.
   B. **Ten to 40 days** from the onset of fever, the most common cause of death in untreated children is myocardial infarction caused by coronary aneurysms. After 40 days, healing and stenosis of the post-aneurysmal coronary artery develops.

III. **Clinical manifestations**
   A. **Abrupt onset of high but remittent fever** between 38 and 41 degrees C is characteristic of KS.
   B. **Within 2 to 5 days, the child develops other diagnostic signs of KS:** Conjunctival injection, mouth changes, an erythematous rash, changes in the hands and feet, and unilateral cervical lymphadenopathy.
   C. **Eye involvement** consists of conjunctival injection and photophobia.
   D. **The lips** are initially bright red, progressing over 3 days to swelling, cracking, and bleeding. Prominent papillae on the tongue create a strawberry appearance, and the oral cavity and pharynx is diffusely erythematous.
   E. **The skin rash** is deeply erythematous with slightly raised margins, varying in size from 2 to 3 mm papules to large plaques covering several centimeters. The rash often is urticarial and may be intensely pruritic. The rash frequently affects the face, often forming a mask-like area around the eyes, nose, and mouth. It may be distributed more prominently on the trunk or on the extremities.
   F. **Firm, indurative edema of the hands and feet** and diffuse red-purple discoloration of palms and soles develop. The edema is sharply demarcated at the wrists and

around the sides of the hands and feet.

G. **Cervical lymph node involvement** occurs in 50% of patients, manifesting as sudden onset of a firm swelling on one side of the neck.

H. **Ten to 20 days after the onset of fever**, in early convalescence, desquamation starts just under the fingernails and toenails and proceeds to involve the entire palm and sole.

Kawasaki Syndrome: Diagnostic Criteria

I. **Fever** for ≥ 5 days (usually >102°F)
II. **At least four of five features**
   A. Bilateral conjunctival injection
   B. Cervical adenitis (unilateral ≥ 1.5 cm diameter, non-fluctuant)
   C. Rash (truncal, perineal accentuation, polymorphous but non-vesicular)
   D. Inflamed oral mucosae (fissured lips, strawberry tongue)
   E. Hand and feet inflammation (periungual peeling around 14-21 days)
III. No alternate diagnosis
IV. Fever plus 3/5 criteria are diagnostic when coronary abnormalities are present

---

IV. **Associated features**
   A. **Extreme irritability and emotional lability** is common.
   B. **Mild cerebrospinal fluid pleocytosis** occurs in 25%. The CSF cell count is between 50 and 150/mm³ and is mononuclear. Protein levels are normal to slightly elevated, and glucose level is normal.
   C. **Urethritis** is present in 60% and is characterized by sterile pyuria. Red blood cells may be detected.
   D. **Severe abdominal pain** occurs in 20% in the first few days, and it may be associated with elevated amylase and lipase levels.
   E. **Liver involvement** occurs in 40%; 10% have a bilirubin level >2 mg/dL. The direct fraction is elevated.
   F. **Cardiac manifestations**
      1. Tachycardia with gallop rhythm is present in 60%, and congestive heart failure occurs in 20%. Thirty percent have a pericardial effusion, and 30% have tricuspid insufficiency.
      2. Prolongation of the PR interval and first-degree heart block are very common, but more significant arrhythmias are rare. Coronary artery aneurysms develop in 18-25%.

V. **Differential diagnosis**
   A. The differential diagnosis includes staphylococcal toxic shock syndrome, scarlatiniform erythroderma, streptococcal scarlet fever, staphylococcal scalded skin syndrome, measles, febrile viral exanthems, hypersensitivity reactions (Stevens-Johnson syndrome), and juvenile rheumatoid arthritis.
   B. KS should be considered in all young children who have a fever of unknown origin, or fever and severe lymphadenopathy, rash, conjunctival injection, hand and feet changes, and mouth changes.

VI. **Laboratory findings**
   A. Erythrocyte sedimentation rate, C-reactive protein, and alpha-1-antitrypsin are elevated. White blood cell (WBC) **count is elevated**, with a polymorphonuclear cell predominance. Bacterial cultures should be drawn to exclude bacterial infection.
   B. Platelet counts are elevated, peaking at 650,000-2,000,000/mm³ between days

10-20.
C. Mild-to-moderate anemia usually is present. Bilirubin is elevated in 10%, and liver enzymes are moderately elevated in the first week in 40%. Hypoalbuminemia is common. Urinalysis shows pyuria in 60%.

VII. **Treatment of Kawasaki syndrome**
   A. **Intravenous gamma globulin.** As soon as KS is diagnosed, a baseline echocardiogram is obtained and IVIG 2 g/kg is given in an 8- to 12-hour infusion. Heart rate and blood pressure should be monitored during the infusion.
   B. **Aspirin.** High-dose aspirin therapy is started on the same day as IVIG. The aspirin dosage is 100 mg/kg/day until a few days after defervescence or until the 14th day of illness. This is followed by a daily dose of 3 to 5 mg/kg until the ESR and platelet counts return to normal, usually after 8 weeks.
   C. **Cardiac evaluation and monitoring**
      1. Serial echocardiograms should monitor the coronary arteries, valves, and ventricles.
      2. Electrocardiography is useful in the acute stage to evaluate heart block or myocarditis, QRS amplitude reduction, T wave changes, or QT interval changes.

VIII. **Prognosis.** KS usually is self-limited; however, cardiac damage may be serious. Twenty percent of all patients not treated with IVIG develop coronary artery aneurysms, appearing 7 days to 4 weeks after the onset of KS.

References, see page 164.

Juvenile Rheumatoid Arthritis

Juvenile rheumatoid arthritis (JRA) is the most common rheumatic condition in children. Between 5 and 18 of every 100,000 children develop JRA each year; the overall prevalence is approximately 30 to 150 per 100,000. The course of JRA can be highly variable: some patients recover fully, whereas others experience lifelong symptoms and significant disability.

I. **Clinical manifestations**
   A. The inflammation of JRA targets the synovial tissue. Affected joints are swollen, limited in motion, stiff, painful, warm, and occasionally erythematous. The etiology of JRA is unknown. Immune complex disease may perpetuate the synovitis. If synovitis persists, structures of the joint will be permanently damaged.
   B. There are three subgroups of JRA: systemic-onset disease, polyarticular-onset disease, and pauciarticular-onset disease. Extraarticular manifestations include the iridocyclitis, rheumatoid nodules; fever, rash, polyserositis, hepatosplenomegaly, lymphadenopathy, anemia, leukocytosis, myocarditis, interstitial lung disease, disseminated intravascular coagulation, and amyloidosis. Growth retardation may occur with chronic JRA.
   C. Diagnosis of JRA usually requires onset of disease during childhood, presence of chronic synovitis, and exclusion of other diseases.

Objective Signs of Arthritis	
Joint Swelling - Synovial hypertrophy - Increased amounts of synovial fluid - Swelling of periarticular tissues **Joint Pain** - On motion - On palpation (tenderness) - At rest	**Loss of Joint Motion** - Stiffness of joints **Joint Warmth** **Joint Erythema**

II. Laboratory studies

A. There are no diagnostic laboratory tests for JRA. Acute phase reactants such as the erythrocyte sedimentation rate and C-reactive protein generally are elevated.

B. Standard radiographs are not diagnostic of early JRA. Joint destruction may occur in late JRA. Such late changes include narrowing of the "joint space," erosions of subchondral or juxtaarticular bone, and joint destruction. Early changes include osteoporosis, periostitis, and soft-tissue swelling.

American College of Rheumatology Criteria for Diagnosis of JRA
Diagnostic Requirements For JRA • Documented arthritis of one or more joints for 6 weeks or longer • Exclusion of other conditions associated with childhood arthritis - Other rheumatic diseases - Infectious diseases - Childhood malignancies - Nonrheumatic conditions of bones and joints - Miscellaneous conditions

III. Treatment of juvenile rheumatoid arthritis

A. First-line therapy includes nonsteroidal antiinflammatory drugs (NSAIDs). In addition, intra-articular corticosteroid injections have been shown to be safe and effective and may have beneficial effects on growth parameters. Physical therapy is important for reducing pain and maintaining joint and muscle function.

B. **NSAIDs.** Conventional NSAIDs inhibit both the cyclooxygenase (COX)-1 form of the enzyme, which releases prostaglandins that protect the stomach and kidneys, and the COX-2 inducible form, which produces prostaglandins involved in the inflammatory process.

NSAID Treatment of Juvenile Rheumatoid Arthritis	
Ibuprofen (Motrin)	*1 to 12 years:* 10 mg/kg PO q 4 to 6 h *More than 12 years:* 200 to 400 mg PO q 4 h; maximum dose 1,200 mg/day
Naproxen (Aleve)	5 mg/kg PO q 12 h; maximum dose 750 mg/day

C. **Disease-Modifying Antirheumatic Drugs.** The term "disease-modifying antirheumatic drugs" (DMARD) is limited to agents that retard radiologic progression of disease.

1. **Methotrexate**
   a. Methotrexate is currently the most frequently used DMARD for JRA. Between 60% and 80% of JRA patients experience some clinical improvement.

      b. The most common adverse events are gastrointestinal symptoms, which occur in 13% of patients. Liver toxicity does not seem to be a major concern in pediatric patients; blood counts and transaminases should be checked every 4 to 8 weeks.

   2. Sulfasalazine. Sulfasalazine is significantly more effective than placebo in suppressing disease activity. However, drug toxicity is a problem. Blood counts and transaminase levels should be monitored.

D. New drugs for juvenile rheumatoid arthritis

   1. Etanercept (Embrel) is approved for use in reducing signs and symptoms and delaying structural damage in patients with moderately to severely active adult RA, and for reducing signs and symptoms of moderately to severely active polyarticular-course JRA that is refractory to 1 or more DMARDs. Etanercept should be reserved until after methotrexate failure in JRA.

   2. COX-2 inhibitors. A new class of therapeutic NSAID agents has been designed to inhibit selectively the COX-2 enzyme. Celecoxib and rofecoxib are associated with a lower incidence of ulcers than conventional NSAIDs. COX-2 inhibitors may be helpful in patients who experience gastrointestinal adverse events.

References, see page 164.

Renal and Urologic Disorders

Hematuria

Hematuria occurs in about 0.5% and 1% of all children. It is defined as more than
to 10 RBCs per high-power microscopic field from a centrifuged midstream voided urin
sample. The urine may be yellow, pink, red, brown, or smoky. Hemoglobin and myoglobi
will produce the same color changes on the dipstick as intact RBCs. Each urine sampl
that tests positive for blood by dipstick must be examined microscopically to confirr
the presence of intact RBCs.

I. Clinical evaluation
   A. If microscopic hematuria has been present for 1 month or more, further investigatio
      for the cause is indicated. Vigorous exercise such as jogging or bike riding ma
      cause hematuria. Abdominal, back or flank pain, especially when associated wit
      bruising, suggests child abuse. Dysuria, urinary frequency, and suprapubic pai
      or tenderness suggests a urinary tract infection or hypercalciuria.
   B. Abdominal pain may be associated with an abdominal mass, nephrolithiasis, c
      Henoch-Schönlein purpura. Aspirin, non-steroidal anti-inflammatory agents, antibiotics
      methyldopa, and other drugs can cause hematuria.
   C. A history of edema, hypertension, skin rash, pallor, joint swelling or tenderness
      abdominal pain, or bloody diarrhea suggests postinfectious glomerulonephritis
      Henoch-Schönlein purpura, lupus nephritis, hemolytic uremic syndrome, or immunoglobuli
      (Ig) A nephropathy.
   D. If sore throat or pyoderma precedes the hematuria by 7 to 30 days, poststreptococca
      acute glomerulonephritis must be ruled out. Hematuria with a concurrent uppe
      respiratory infection strongly suggests IgA nephropathy. Each of these forms c
      glomerulonephritis usually is associated with proteinuria and RBC casts.

Evaluation of Hematuria

Patient history, family history, physical examination
Examination of urine for red blood cell casts and crystals
Screening for proteinuria with a dipstick
Examination of urine of first-degree relatives for hematuria
Urine culture
Urinary calcium/urinary creatinine; 24-hour urinary calcium excretion
Serum creatinine, C3, streptozyme titer
Renal ultrasonography
Plain abdominal film if nephrolithiasis is suspected

Differential Diagnosis of Persistent Hematuria	
Without Proteinuria	**With Proteinuria**
Urinary tract infection	Urinary tract infection
Hypercalciuria	Poststreptococcal acute glomerulonephritis
Thin basement membrane disease	IgA nephropathy
Sickle cell disease or trait	Henoch-Schönlein purpura
Renal cystic disease	Membranoproliferative glomerulonephritis
Nephrolithiasis	Lupus nephritis
Renal anatomic abnormalities	Alport syndrome Hemolytic-uremic syndrome Other forms of glomerulonephritis

E. A family history of hematuria without renal failure may be seen with thin basement membrane disease. A family history of hematuria, chronic renal failure, dialysis or renal transplantation with bilateral deafness and ocular abnormalities suggests Alport syndrome. An audiogram is indicated for children suspected of having Alport syndrome.

F. A family history of nephrolithiasis raises the diagnostic possibility of nephrolithiasis or hypercalciuria. A family history of autosomal dominant polycystic kidney disease requires that this disease be ruled out by ultrasound. Sickle cell disease or sickle cell trait in the patient's family may suggest this diagnosis.

G. **Urinalysis.** RBCs from areas of the urinary tract other than glomeruli will be normal in size with smooth edges (eumorphic). Nonglomerular bleeding usually is associated with normal urinary protein excretion and an absence of RBC casts.

Familial Causes of Hematuria

Polycystic kidney disease
Thin basement membrane disease
Sickle cell disease or trait
Alport syndrome (hereditary nephritis with deafness)
Hypercalciuria with family history of nephrolithiasis

H. Preliminary tests should include a urine culture, blood sickle cell preparation in African-American children, urinary calcium; urinary creatinine ratio, serum creatinine; C3, and streptozyme titer. Ultrasonography of the kidneys and urinary bladder is recommended to rule out polycystic kidney disease, tumor, ureteropelvic junction obstruction, and stones.

I. The presence of proteinuria (>1+ on dipstick) strongly suggests glomerulonephritis. The diagnosis of glomerulonephritis demands microscopic inspection of the urinary sediment for RBC casts. RBCs that have bizarre shapes, blebs, or burrs (dysmorphic RBCs) correlate with a glomerular origin of the RBC.

J. **Proteinuria**
   1. If proteinuria is present on urinalysis, urinary protein excretion should be measured by a timed 12- or 24-hour urine collection or a urine protein:urine creatinine

ratio on a single voided sample.
2. A complete blood count, C3, C4, antistreptolysin-O titer, streptozyme titer, serum electrolytes, blood urea nitrogen, serum creatinine, serum albumin, test for lupus erythematosus, hepatitis B screen, and antinuclear cytoplasmic antibody titer are indicated to clarify the type of glomerulonephritis. A screening urinalysis on first-degree family members is also important. When confirmatory serologic tests are nondiagnostic, a renal biopsy usually is indicated.

Renal Structural Abnormalities Associated with Hematuria

Polycystic kidney disease
Ureteropelvic junction obstruction
Vesicoureteral reflux
Renal or bladder stones, diverticula or tumors
Renal arteriovenous fistula
Foreign bodies

References, see page 164.

Fluids and Electrolytes

Disorders affecting the body fluids and electrolytes are treated by supplying maintenance requirements, correcting volume and electrolyte deficits, and by replacing ongoing abnormal losses.

I. Dehydration
   A. Maintenance fluid and electrolytes
      1. Sensible losses, primarily urinary, account for 50% of daily fluid requirements. Caloric requirements for growth can be estimated as equivalent on a kcal-for-mL basis to water requirements.
      2. Factors that increase the requirements for calories and water are fever (10% for each degree), physical activity, ongoing gastrointestinal losses, hyperventilation and hypermetabolic states.

Maintenance Requirements for Fluid and Electrolytes

Body Weight	0 to 10 kg	10 to 20 kg	>20 kg
Water Volume	100 mL/kg	1000 mL + 50 mL/kg for each kg >10 kg	1500 mL + 20 mL/kg for each kg >20 kg
Sodium	3 mEq/kg	3 mEq/kg	3 mEq/kg
Potassium	2 mEq/kg	2 mEq/kg	2 mEq/kg
Chloride	5 mEq/kg	5 mEq/kg	5 mEq/kg

      3. Abnormal losses, such as those arising from nasogastric aspiration, prolonged diarrhea or burns, should be measured, and replaced on a volume for volume basis.
   B. Estimation of deficit
      1. Estimation of volume depletion should assess fever, vomiting, diarrhea, and urine output. Recent feeding, including type and volume of food and drink,

and weight change should be determined.

Estimation of Dehydration

Degree of Dehydration	Mild	Moderate	Severe
Weight Loss--Infants	5%	10%	15%
Weight Loss--Children	3-4%	6-8%	10%
Pulse	Normal	Slightly increased	Very increased
Blood Pressure	Normal	Normal to orthostatic, >10 mm Hg change	Orthostatic to shock
Behavior	Normal	Irritable	Hyperirritable to lethargic
Thirst	Slight	Moderate	Intense
Mucous Membranes	Normal	Dry	Parched
Tears	Present	Decreased	Absent tears, sunken eyes
Anterior Fontanelle	Normal	Normal to sunken	Sunken
External Jugular Vein	Visible when supine	Not visible except with supraclavicular pressure	Not visible even with supraclavicular pressure
Skin	Capillary refill <2 sec	Delayed capillary refill, 2-4 sec (decreased turgor)	Very delayed capillary refill (>4 sec), tenting; cool, acrocyanotic or mottled skin
Urine Specific Gravity (SG)	>1.020	>1.020; oliguria	Oliguria or anuria

2. The percent dehydration is used to calculate the milliliters of body water deficit per kilogram of body weight.

C. **Isonatremic dehydration**
1. The most common cause of dehydration in infants is diarrhea. Children who have a brief illness and anorexia usually present with isotonic dehydration.
2. **Oral rehydration**
   a. Moderate volume depletion should be treated with oral fluids. The majority of patients who have gastroenteritis can be treated with oral rehydration therapy.
   b. Small aliquots of oral hydration solution (Ricelyte, Pedialyte, Resol, Rehydralyte) are given as tolerated to provide 50 mL/kg over 4 hours in mild dehydration, and up to 100 mL/kg over 6 hours in moderate dehydration. Once rehydration is accomplished, maintenance fluid is given at 100 mL/kg per day.
3. **Parenteral rehydration**
   a. Parenteral fluids should be given for severe volume depletion, altered states of consciousness, intractable vomiting, and abdominal distention or ileus.
   b. The first phase of treatment rapidly expands the vascular volume. Intravenous

normal saline or Ringers lactate (10-20 mL/kg) should be given over
hour.

c. The next phase of treatment is aimed at correcting the deficit, providing
maintenance, and replacing ongoing abnormal losses. In severe depletion
half of the calculated deficit is given over the first 8 hours and the second
half over the next 16 hours; maintenance needs are provided. Five percent
glucose should be used as the stock solution and NaCl is added according
to the estimated need.

d. Children who have isonatremic dehydration require 8 to 10 mEq of Na
per kg of body weight for repletion of deficit and 3 mEq/kg per day for
maintenance. This Na^+ is given in a volume consisting of the calculated
maintenance for water and the estimated water deficit. Once urine flow
occurs, KCl is added at a concentration of 20 mEq/L.

D. Hyponatremia and hyponatremic dehydration

1. The signs and symptoms of hyponatremia correlate with the rapidity and
extent of the fall in serum Na^+ concentration. Symptoms include apathy, nausea
vomiting, cramps, weakness, headache, seizures, and coma.

2. If the correction of fluid and electrolyte losses is excessively rapid, the brain
may sustain injury. In severe hyponatremia, plasma Na^+ concentration should
be corrected at no more than 10-12 mEq/L/day.

3. **Differential diagnosis of hyponatremia**

   a. **Hypovolemia**

      (1) The most frequent cause of hypovolemic hyponatremia is viral gastroenteritis
      with vomiting and diarrhea. Other causes of hypovolemic hyponatremia
      include percutaneous losses or third space sequestration of fluid (ascites
      burns, peritonitis).

      (2) Renal sodium loss (urinary Na^+ >20 mEq/L) may be caused by diuretics
      salt-wasting nephropathy, proximal renal tubular acidosis, and lack
      of or resistance to mineralocorticoid.

   b. **Euvolemia.** The most common cause of euvolemic hyponatremia is the
   syndrome of inappropriate antidiuretic hormone secretion, which is caused
   by water retention (urinary Na^+ is usually >20 mEq/L). Causes include
   tumors, pulmonary disorders, CNS infection, and certain drugs. Euvolemic
   hyponatremia may also occur in infants fed excessively diluted infant formula.

   c. **Hypervolemia.** Hypervolemic hyponatremia, associated with edema
   may result from water retention and excess Na^+, as in nephrosis, congestive
   heart failure, cirrhosis, or renal failure.

4. **Management of hyponatremia**

   a. Hypovolemic patients who have hyponatremia first require volume repletion
   with normal saline, then a solution containing salt is given to correct the
   Na^+ deficit (10 to 12 mEq/kg of body weight or 15 mEq/kg in severe hyponatremia
   and to provide the Na^+ maintenance needs (3 mEq/kg per day) in a 5%
   dextrose solution.

   b. For a serum Na^+ concentration of 120 to 130 mEq/L, this amount should
   be given over a 24-hour period. For a serum Na^+ concentration <120 mEq/L
   the rehydration should be spread out over several days at a rate of 10
   mEq/day.

   c. **Symptomatic hyponatremia** (headache, lethargy, disorientation) requires
   urgent therapy to prevent seizures or coma.

      (1) Hypertonic saline (3% saline solution) should be used to raise the
      serum Na^+ by 1 to 2 mEq/L per hour or halfway toward normal during
      the first 8 hours.

      (2) A correction using 3% saline over 4 hours can be calculated according

to the following formula:

Sodium deficit in mEq = (125 - observed [Na^+]) x body weight in kg x 0.6

E. Hypernatremia and hypernatremic dehydration

1. The hypernatremic patient is usually also dehydrated. Total body Na^+ most commonly is decreased. Affected patients frequently exhibit lethargy or confusion, muscle twitching, hyperreflexia, or convulsions. Fever is common, and the skin may feel thickened or doughy.

2. **Differential diagnosis**
   a. Diarrhea, which usually results in isonatremic or hyponatremic dehydration, may cause hypernatremia in the presence of persistent fever, anorexia, vomiting, and decreased fluid intake.
   b. Other causes of hypernatremia include water and Na^+ deficit from skin losses or renal losses, and water losses from central or nephrogenic diabetes insipidus (DI) or drugs (lithium, cyclophosphamide).

3. **Management**
   a. Initial therapy requires administration of normal saline or Ringers lactate to restore circulating plasma volume. Hypovolemic patients who have hypernatremia require a hypotonic solution containing salt to restore the Na^+ deficit (2-5 mEq/kg of body weight) and to provide the Na^+ maintenance (3 mEq/kg of Na^+) in a solution containing 20-40 mmol/L of KCl and 5% glucose.
   b. For a serum Na^+ concentration of 150-160 mEq/L, this volume should be given over 24-hours. An elevated serum Na^+ concentration should be corrected by no more than 10 mEq/L per day.
   c. For a serum Na^+ concentration >160 mEq/L, the rehydration should be spread out over several days to lower the Na^+ concentration to 150 mEq/L by 10 mEq/day.

Potassium disorders

A. Hypokalemia

1. Hypokalemia (serum K^+ concentration <3 mEq/L) is most frequently caused by gastrointestinal K^+ losses or renal losses (nasogastric suction, protracted vomiting, diuretics, renal tubular disease). Manifestations of hypokalemia include arrhythmias, neuromuscular excitability (hyporeflexia or paralysis, decreased peristalsis, ileus), and rhabdomyolysis.

2. Intracellular K^+ concentration can be estimated from the electrocardiogram, which may reveal flattened T waves, shortened P-R interval and QRS complex, and eventually U waves.

3. **Management**
   a. In the presence of cardiac arrhythmias, extreme muscle weakness, or respiratory distress, patients should receive KCl intravenously with cardiac monitoring. Once the serum K^+ is stabilized, oral administration is preferable.
   b. If the patient is likely to be hypophosphatemic, a phosphate salt should be used. In metabolic alkalosis, KCl should be used; in renal tubular acidosis, a citrate salt should be used.

B. Hyperkalemia

1. The most common cause of hyperkalemia (K^+ >5.5 mEq/L) is "pseudohyperkalemia" from hemolysis of the blood sample. This cause should be excluded by repeating the measurement on a free-flowing venous sample. Children may display hyperkalemia in metabolic acidosis, tissue catabolism, renal failure, volume depletion, or hypoaldosteronism.

2. In salt-losing congenital adrenal hyperplasia, due to complete deficiency

of the enzyme 21-hydroxylase, the symptoms in affected male infants appear in the first weeks of life and include dehydration and failure to thrive together with low serum Na^+ and high K^+ concentrations. Affected female infants usually are diagnosed at birth because of ambiguous genitalia.

3. Manifestations of hyperkalemia include cardiac arrhythmias, paresthesias, muscle weakness, and paralysis.

4. The electrocardiogram demonstrates narrow, peaked T waves and shortened QT intervals at K^+ concentrations >6 mEq/L and depressed ST segment and widened QRS complex at K^+ concentrations >8 mEq/L.

5. **Management**
   a. Emergent therapy to reverse potentially life-threatening hyperkalemia consists of intravenous calcium. The onset of action is rapid; however the duration is less than 30 minutes.
   b. Emergent administration of glucose will cause K^+ to redistribute to the intracellular space. Glucose, 0.5 gm/kg, can be given over 30-60 minutes when EKG changes are present.
   c. Sodium polystyrene sulfonate (Kayexalate) (1 gm/kg) can be given by high-rectal enema or orally. Severe hyperkalemia is treated with hemodialysis.

III. Acid-base disorders
   A. The pH of the body fluids normally is between 7.35 and 7.45.
   B. **Metabolic acidosis**
      1. Acidosis results from the addition of acid or the removal of alkali from body fluids, and it causes a compensatory increase in ventilation (respiratory alkalosis) and a fall in pCO_2. Manifestations of acidosis include depressed myocardial contractility, arrhythmias, hypotension, and pulmonary edema.
      2. **Diagnosis**
         a. Addition of a fixed acid to the extracellular fluid causes the formation of unmeasured anions. These unmeasured anions are referred to as the anion gap, which can be estimated as:

         $$\text{Anion gap} = Na^+ - (Cl^- + HCO_3^-) = 10\text{-}12 \text{ mEq/L}$$

      3. **Differential diagnosis**
         a. **Normal anion gap (hyperchloremic) acidosis**
            (1) This disorder occurs when HCO_3^- is lost from the body, either through the gastrointestinal tract or the kidneys. Diarrheal fluid is high in HCO_3^-, high in K^+, and low in Cl^-. Thus, diarrhea causes hypokalemia and hyperchloremic acidosis.
            (2) Failure to excrete acid occurs in mild chronic renal insufficiency and RTA.
         b. **Increased anion gap acidosis** may be caused by diabetic ketoacidosis, lactic acidosis, ingestion of toxins (aspirin, ethylene glycol), and renal failure.
      4. **Treatment of acidosis**
         a. Bicarbonate should be given when plasma HCO_3^- is <5 mmol/L. Bicarbonate should be added to a hypotonic solution and given as a continuous infusion over 1 hour. The amount to infuse is calculated with the following formula:

         $$\text{Amount to infuse in mEq} = \text{weight in kg } (15 - \text{observed } [HCO_3^-]) \times 0.5$$

         b. With severe watery diarrhea, resulting in moderate-to-severe metabolic acidosis, volume replacement is the primary mode of therapy.

C. Metabolic alkalosis

1. Alkalosis results from a gain of base or a loss of acid. The common clinical manifestations are lethargy, confusion, neuromuscular irritability, arrhythmias, and seizures.

2. **Differential diagnosis**
   a. Causes of metabolic alkalosis include alkali administration, vomiting, and nasogastric aspiration. In patients with GI loss of acid from vomiting, urinary Cl^- concentration is usually below 20 mEq/L.
   b. Cushing syndrome, Bartter syndrome or primary aldosteronism may cause metabolic alkalosis.

3. **Treatment**
   a. Therapy consists of identifying and treating the underlying pathology.
   b. In mild-to-moderate alkalosis, provision of Cl^- will allow the kidney to excrete the excess base.

D. Respiratory acidosis

1. Respiratory acidosis is induced by an increase in pCO_2 which lowers plasma pH. Causes of respiratory acidosis include airway obstruction, and pulmonary disorders.

2. Treatment consists of mechanical ventilation and correction of the underlying disorder.

E. Respiratory alkalosis

1. Respiratory alkalosis is caused by a decrease in pCO_2, secondary to hyperventilation, resulting in dizziness, confusion, and seizures.

2. Causes of respiratory alkalosis include hyperventilation caused by CNS disorders and panic disorder. Treatment involves correcting the underlying disorder. Rebreathing into a bag may decrease the severity of symptoms.

References, see page 164.

Vesicoureteral Reflux

Vesicoureteral reflux is defined as the retrograde flow of urine from the bladder into the ureter and collecting system. Children who have a urinary tract infection (UTI) have 45% incidence of vesicoureteral reflux. The incidence increases with decreasing age, and 65% of patients are females. In a male who has a UTI, the risk of reflux is 30%.

Diagnosis

A. **Radiologic evaluation** for vesicoureteral reflux should be undertaken when a urinary tract infection occurs in one of the following patients:
1. UTI in a male.
2. UTI in an infant (under two years of age).
3. Pyelonephritis in a female.
4. Recurrent UTI in a female.

B. Evaluation of children who have prenatally diagnosed hydronephrosis consists of a postnatal renal ultrasonography (RUS) and voiding cystourethrogram (VCUG). These patients initially are managed nonoperatively because a significant number of children will stop refluxing within the first 2 years of life.

C. The radiologic evaluation of the child who has had a febrile UTI includes a voiding cystourethrogram and renal ultrasonography. The radiologic evaluation should be performed after diagnosing the first UTI. If the child who has a UTI is toxic and has been hospitalized, the renal ultrasonography should be obtained after admission. The VCUG should be performed as soon as the urine is sterile.

D. **Grading of vesicoureteral reflux**
1. **Grade I reflux** is defined as retrograde urine flow into a non-dilated ureter
2. **Grade II reflux** refers to the filling of a non-dilated ureter and a non-dilated renal pelvis.
3. **Grade III reflux** consists of mild dilatation of the collecting system, but the fornices remain sharp.
4. **Grade IV reflux** consists of moderate dilation and blunted fornices.
5. **Grade V reflux** is defined as massive dilatation and tortuosity of the collecting system.

II. Medical management

A. Most cases of vesicoureteral reflux are managed nonoperatively with attention to perineal hygiene, normalization of bowel and voiding habits, and prophylactic antibiotics.

B. Diaper rashes and chemical irritants such as bubble bath should be discouraged because they predispose to UTIs. Children should avoid harsh soaps, shampoos and tub baths. If constipation is a problem, stool softeners and scheduled defecation programs are effective.

C. **Prophylactic antibiotics**
1. Trimethoprim/sulfamethoxazole is the most commonly used drug, given in a dose of 2 mg/kg of trimethoprim plus 10mg/kg of sulfamethoxazole, orally once a day before bedtime. For the newborn, amoxicillin is preferred for prophylaxis.
2. Suppression continues until the reflux resolves spontaneously or until surgery is performed.

D. **Patient monitoring**
1. Urine cultures are obtained monthly for 3 months after any UTI. Thereafter a urine culture is obtained every other month for 6 months. If the urine remain sterile, surveillance cultures are then obtained every 3 months.
2. Repeat imaging is obtained every 6-12 months. Follow-up can be done with a nuclear cystogram. Patients who have minimal or no scarring may only need an ultrasound.
3. **Grade I and II vesicoureteral reflux** is followed on low-dose antibiotic chemoprophylaxis. The reflux resolves in most children.
4. **Grades III and IV** reflux generally are managed nonoperatively initially.
5. **Grade V vesicoureteral reflux**, except neonates, is treated with surgery at diagnosis because this grade of reflux, especially if bilateral, has a very low likelihood of spontaneous resolution.

References
References for this book can be obtained at www.ccspublishing.com/ccs.

Index